Y0-BDG-289

Doulas' Guide to Birthing Your Way

Jan S. Mallak, 2LAS, ICCE-CD-CPD-IAT, CD-PCD(DONA), CPD(CAPPA)

Teresa F. Bailey, J.D., M.L.S., CD(DONA), LLL Leader

Doulas' Guide to Birthing Your Way

Jan S. Mallak, 2LAS, ICCE-CD-CPD-IAT, CD-PCD(DONA), CPD(CAPPA)

Teresa F. Bailey, J.D., M.L.S., CD(DONA), LLL Leader

© Copyright 2010 by Jan S. Mallak and Teresa F. Bailey

Hale Publishing, L.P.

1712 N. Forest St.

Amarillo, TX 79106-7017

806-376-9900

800-378-1317

www.iBreastfeeding.com

www.hale-publishing.com

All rights reserved. No part of this publication may be reproduced or transmitted in any form or by any means, electronic or mechanical, including photocopy, recording, stored in a database or any information storage, or put into a computer, without prior written permission from the publisher.

Library of Congress Control Number: 2009943969

ISBN-13: 978-0-9823379-7-4

Printed in Canada.

Table of Contents

By Dr. John Kennell, world-renowned pediatrician and co-founder of DONA International (Doulas of North America). He is also coauthor of *The Doula Book*.

This describes how the book is *different* and what it will do for *you*, the mother, preparing for your birth (or the doula hired to help you). Doula techniques can help any birthing mother, not just first-time moms. This book guides you through discovering your own birth vision.

Where you give birth is not nearly as important as who is there. The *human environment*—the people who surround you and your relationships with them—is what sets the tone for your birth, directly affecting its safety and success, as well as your own satisfaction.

Spiritual, mediatorial, physical, emotional, informational—these are the five kinds of support you will need to be able to make the right choices for your birth. Taking all these aspects of the experience into account helps you have the confidence to stay in control.

You can't *plan* a birth—birth is a natural event. But a birth vision communicates your philosophy, preferences, and priorities to everyone on the birth team in a way that's easy to understand.

Now is the time to build your relationships with your birth team. It's also the time to learn what you need to know to make the right choices, to put together your birth bag to take with you, and to prepare your body for its birth task.

Now that you know what to expect before, during, and after your birth, you have the information you need to put together your own birth vision. Here are worksheets and examples to help you put your philosophy, preferences, and priorities on paper.

To Zeev, my bright-eyed grandson who made me love birth even more—J.S.M.

To Simon, who taught me the important job of mothering—T.F.B.

Acknowledgments

We would like to express our profound appreciation to Dr. Jack Newman for reading and offering assistance on our breastfeeding chapter. We also wish to thank Dr. John Kennell for writing the foreword and his support in the doula spirit. We would also like to thank The Midwife Center in Pittsburgh for letting us use their facilities for photo sessions and writing.

We would like to express our deep appreciation for the support we received from both of our families, with special thanks to Christopher Bailey for help with editing and photography, Heather Mallak for her illustrations, and Dror Yaron for photographs. The encouragement from our families was invaluable.

We would also like to thank "Heart and Hands" doulas and clients for modeling for our photos. And special thanks to our doula clients who inspired us to write this book. We truly appreciate the honor of being able to attend their births and share in the true labor of love that birth is. These special people have influenced us and supported us during our rite of passage into the publishing world.

Foreword

This well-written new book, *Doulas' Guide to Birthing Your Way* by Jan Mallak and Teresa Bailey, contains a wealth of information for pregnant women and their partners. Jan Mallak was just starting her career as a childbirth educator at the time the report about the doula was published in the *New England Journal of Medicine*. This article described the beneficial effects of continuous support during labor by a woman Dr. Marshall Klaus and I called a "doula."

Jan's early doula activities have expanded to coordinating a group of 17 doulas called the "Heart and Hands" Doula Service, providing birth and postpartum support since 1995. The co-author, Teresa Bailey, is a lawyer who has given up her law career to become a doula. She is also a leader in the breastfeeding organization La Leche League. They have written this book, *Doulas' Guide to Birthing Your Way*, for both expectant mothers and for doulas. Combining the two is a wise decision, I believe. It enhances the woman-to-woman connection that can be a powerful force during and after childbirth. Both Jan and Teresa have now served as doulas over and over again for mothers delivering in the 21st century, a period characterized by much greater use of obstetric interventions and increased necessity for continuous support for all mothers by a knowledgeable, experienced doula. The authors have written this book "to encourage women to think about, create, and believe in their own personal vision of birth." And they present "tips, tools, and techniques" to help women meet the birth task with more confidence. In the busy life of working couples in the United States, there does not seem to be time for pregnant women and their partners to think about, discuss, and plan many aspects of their labor and delivery and what will happen in the minutes, hours, and days that follow. The book's quizzes, checklists, birth vision suggestions, mother's and partner's activity pages, and choices in childbirth, and other extra features will provide valuable advance preparation for the expectant parents, and for doulas, also.

The story at the beginning of the first chapter describes the birthing experience for hundreds and thousands of mothers in the U.S. from the eighteenth to the beginning of the twentieth century. One or more women who usually had previous experience with labor and delivery were present with the laboring woman, providing advice, encouragement, and physical support. Often these were women the pregnant woman knew and trusted, such as her mother, sister, or a close friend. To gain some perspective, it is probable that support or the presence of a woman with another woman during labor has been the almost universal human practice, starting 400,000 to 500,000 years ago. That was the time of a revolution in human childbirth. It was when the human brain and head size increased greatly, and at about the same time the human pelvic bones were changing to enable humans to walk on two legs, as we do today. The process of the descent and delivery of the baby was changed radically by this. The baby now had to turn to go through the birth canal, and as a consequence, emerged facing backwards. It became dangerous for the laboring woman to deliver her own infant. Support and assistance by a woman became almost universal. Dana Raphael, whose anthropology dissertation gave us the name "doula," pointed out that in all but one of the 150 cultures a family member or friend remained with a mother during labor and delivery. Subsequent childbirth descriptions by anthropologists based on a sample of 186 non-industrial societies that was geographically, historically, and linguistically representative showed that in less than 2% of world societies the woman routinely gives birth alone. And in only 2% was a woman *allowed* to give birth alone.

One hundred years ago at the beginning of the twentieth century, the delivery scene was the same as in the first chapter. The deliveries were performed by midwives and physicians. The laboring woman was still in familiar surroundings with supportive individuals she knew well. In the first third of the twentieth century, birth moved from the home to the hospital, a strange environment with people the woman did not know. Now in the first decade of the twenty-first century, women in labor still come to unfamiliar environments, with even more strangers, and are admitted to a room with multiple strange sights and sounds, with very busy nurses checking monitors, intravenous fluids, and medications. Those who come with the woman, including the father, are often anxious and ill at ease, inadequately prepared for all they hear, see, and smell, and for decision-making affecting the well-being of his wife or son or daughter.

This book comes at an opportune time. I was fortunate to have multiple opportunities to observe labor and childbirth, and the mother and baby in the postpartum period. As a pediatrician, I had abundant experiences with the infant, toddler, and preschooler. There have been many changes, both positive and negative in the mothers' and fathers' experiences with childbirth and their infants and children. In recent years, I have had concerns that we have exceeded the limits of adaptability for some mothers and fathers to develop the traditionally strong emotional ties to their children in the first year. Studies show that if the attachment of a child to the parent is not secure at one year, it probably won't be later on. That is why I am delighted with this book and all it provides for mothers and fathers in the earliest interactions with their newborn. Based on research related to infants and their parents, particularly in the first year, I appreciate how important the nature and quality of what happens with the mother, father, and newborn during labor and delivery (doula support), the first days and weeks (mother and baby together), and the first year will be. In this book, Jan and Teresa provide you with information about the many advantages of support for the mother and father and the newborn by a doula. You will gain valuable insights from many other treasures of information that the book contains. I want to emphasize that what we have learned about the effects of doula support is paramount for everyone concerned. After reading about the remarkable effects of a doula (and there are no unfavorable effects), you will surely want to have a doula for your delivery and will be eager to share information about this book and the doula with your friends.

An independent international body of experts monitors and reviews all published studies of doula support and selects those that meet strict scientific standards. The fifteen research studies that measure up to these standards show significant benefits for mothers supported continuously by a doula during labor and delivery compared with mothers who did not have a doula. That is, fewer mothers need cesarean (operative) deliveries, or the use of forceps or other interventions to speed up or accomplish the safe birth of the baby.

There are many other benefits of this continuous support. For example, there is the assurance that the doula will not leave the mother, the doula's many comfort measures, her ability to inform the laboring mother about the progress she and the baby are making, to explain what is going on, what lies ahead, what the nurse or doctor said or meant, the support she provides to the father, saying that he can leave at any time, that she will remain continuously and assist him in how best to ease the mother's discomfort.

Somehow the presence and teamwork of a relaxed male partner and a devoted doula result in striking outcomes, above and beyond the faster, easier, less painful obstetric outcome: Doula-supported mothers, in contrast to other mothers after the birth, report more pride in themselves, more positive feelings about their coping ability, and a better over-all labor experience. In almost every study, more doula-supported mothers breastfeed successfully, and with this their infants have fewer illnesses, and their mothers report more frequent pleasurable and relaxed "bonding times" together. Compared to mothers who do not have a doula, these mothers are less likely to become depressed and have greater self-esteem. Another difference of great long-term significance is that, in contrast to other mothers, doula-supported mothers rate their baby as better than a standard baby, more beautiful, clever, and easier to manage.

Another striking outcome is that doula-supported mothers are significantly more satisfied with their male partners in the first weeks (71% compared with 30%). This is a significant positive benefit during the stressful early days and weeks, and beyond. And at the visits to the doctor or nurse practitioner, the new mother will be more likely to praise her husband's support and much less likely to comment that her partner "wasn't helpful" and "didn't know what to do." So, best wishes for rewarding birthing experiences to all who read *Doulas' Guide to Birthing Your Way*. Last of all, I appreciated the logo developed by Jan's daughter.

John H. Kennell, M.D.

Introduction

If you're looking for a book that will help you have a satisfying birth experience, this is the book. Giving birth is something you'll remember for the rest of your life. It's not just a physical process; there's a spiritual and emotional side, too.

What you might not know is that how you *feel* about your birth actually affects the physical outcome. If you feel in control and well supported, you're less likely to need medical interventions. You want to have a positive memory that you can cherish—a memory of feeling empowered and supported. This book will guide you through your birth, so that you can create that joyful, positive memory. It also describes how to get a good start on a healthy, happy relationship with your baby.

This book is different from all the other books about birth you've seen. It's written for you, the birthing mother—and for your doula, too, if you have one. It leads you step by step through the birth process, so you'll know exactly what to expect. It will give you the information you need to take control of your own birth and make it *your* rite of Passage. Whether this is your first child or you are an experienced mother, here's your guide to giving birth *your* way, and having the positive experience you've longed for.

You'll learn:

- The five labor support secrets developed and used by doulas
- How to build a birth team that supports you
- How to write a Birth Vision that reflects your priorities
- How to get organized before the birth happens
- The 10 things that *must* be in your birth bag
- What to do when labor begins
- Tips, tools and techniques to help you have the easiest birth you can have
- How to birth the baby during pushing
- Ways to avoid a cesarean birth or how to accomplish a VBAC (vaginal birth after cesarean)

- How to get breastfeeding off to a good start
- The best ways to avoid postpartum depression

Have a pencil ready because we've included lots of interactive tools you can use to discover your real preferences and build your personal birth vision.

Are you ready? Then let's start by taking a look at what makes your feelings about your birth so important.

Chapter 1
The Human Environment

The mother could feel the baby moving down and out as her urges intensified. The power of the movement scared the woman a bit, but her attendants comforted and reassured her. As the stretching increased, one of the neighbors assisting the midwife placed warm cotton rags on the baby's head while it peek-a-booed in and out.

All the women there were encouraging her onward, as they held her and fanned her sweaty body and told her how wonderfully she was handling the hard work of pushing.

Then, as the mother panted, the baby came out in all its shiny glory.

The mother's sister wrapped the baby in the blanket their mother had knitted and placed the little girl on her mama's bare breast. They all looked on with delight as she took right to nursing. The baby opened her mouth like a baby bird and her mother brought her onto the breast. As she held her new daughter skin-to-skin and tummy-to-tummy, the baby settled into a rhythm of active sucking. It made the new mama so happy and proud.

Afterwards, the grandmother dressed her daughter in a beautiful new gown and brushed her hair 100 times, just like when she was a little girl. Her other sister made her some fennel tea and toast with Aunt Ann's homemade blueberry jelly.

The new mother glowed as all the women in the room treated her like she was queen for a day. She soon forgot the hard parts of labor and just continued to fall in love with little Mary.

As the days went by, the community pitched in to help with errands, meals, and other necessities, so the family could recover and transition into a new life together.

More days passed, and the new mother felt recovered and more ready to mother on her own. She was certain she could do this mama thing just fine—as long as one of the ladies was right down the street to guide and advise her.

Confidence Makes the Difference

A birth very much like this could have happened yesterday, a hundred years ago, a thousand years ago, or ten thousand years ago. In most births in most of the world for most of history, the mother has been attended by a variety of other women who cared for her every need. Knowing that she has that support makes the whole experience of labor less a thing to fear and more a thing to look forward to.

Where you give birth is not nearly as important as who is there. The *human environment*—the people who surround you and your relationships with them—is what sets the tone for the birth, directly affecting its safety and success, as well as your own satisfaction.

Every woman thinks about the birth of her baby, and many women fear it. They fear that there will be pain they won't be able to handle. They fear that the birth won't go the way they expect or plan. They fear the unknown.

There's no question that labor is hard work. It also involves some pain. However, most of the time, most women can cope with the pain, without having to resort to drugs. The key is to feel confident and overcome your fears. Fear increases your perception of pain. So the more confidence you have during labor, the less fear you have. The less you fear it, the less it hurts. Then you can feel confident that you can cope during your labor.

Confidence was just what that traditional sisterhood of support gave a new mother. But for the past three generations, women have given birth mostly in hospitals, with little social support. Birth became more of a medical event than a life event. Even fathers weren't allowed into the labor room until the 1960s.

Now, most hospitals are aware of and have had experience with *doulas*. A doula is a woman who stays with the laboring mother all through her labor, giving her the kind of support she would have gotten from the other members of her family or from the villagers. Since doulas provide no medical care, advice, or interpretations, there should be no confusion about roles in the birthing room. A doula helps the mother approach her birth holistically, drawing on her own inner resources to do what the female body was intended to do. If it does turn out that medical interventions are necessary, a doula keeps her informed, which helps the mother make better decisions.

A doula works at calming a woman's fears of the unknown, like the baby's health, the length of labor, and the amount of pain she might have to endure. Even if you think you've planned your pregnancy, you'll still have fears surrounding the birth—especially if this is your first birth. Will you bond with the baby? Will your new life as a parent overwhelm you? Can you meet your own standards for being a good mother? Fears like these can actually impede your natural rhythm of letting labor happen! And those fears can be increased greatly by the wrong sort of environment, both physical and emotional.

In fact, research shows that a happy mother means a happy baby. Your baby is actually healthier if you feel good about yourself and your baby, and confident about your labor. There are fewer problems with breastfeeding and less chance of your having postpartum depression.

Surprisingly enough, it turns out that doulas are one of the most researched topics in obstetrics today. Since 1980 when the doula movement began, more research has been done on doulas than on epidurals, cesareans, and other medical interventions associated with modern birth.

The results of the studies have all led to the same conclusion. Doulas make for better and more successful births. Having a doula in the room measurably decreases the chance of interventions, like analgesia and anesthesia, instrument deliveries, and cesarean births. No matter where the tests are done or on what populations, the results are similar. In fact, merely having another woman continuously in the room has a measurably beneficial effect on the outcome of the birth. The more involved the labor companion is, the more the mother and her baby benefit. There are better outcomes if the woman feels well cared for and is given the freedom to birth following her own rhythm.

The benefits may go far beyond the birth. The whole experience of labor helps define the new mother and how she handles the work associated with raising children. If you feel confident and in control during your labor—even when things don't go quite the way you expected—you're more likely to feel confident and in control with your new family.

Of course, it's not just the doula who affects your emotional state. Everyone in the room—your partner, family, nurses, midwives, doctors, and technicians—contributes to the human environment. The better your relationship with all of them, the better your birth experience will be.

The human environment can be considered the cornerstone of a satisfying birth experience. Feeling loved, cared for, listened to, protected, and informed by the people surrounding you will make you feel empowered. The resulting self-confidence will help you meet the task of giving birth. First, you will need to develop touch and trust relationships with your support team. Building those critical relationships before the birth is a great investment of your time.

Having a sense of how you may best be able to deal with labor is also important. Planning it can lead to disappointment, but envisioning ways of coping can be beneficial. Attending classes, reading books, and going to support group meetings are ways to educate yourself about your choices, so that you can create your own birth vision.

Going to classes with your partner to learn about your body and its innate natural resources will also build your confidence. Knowing tips, tools, and techniques to help you from the beginning to the end of birth will further empower you. Having information and skills to better handle the pain and anxiety associated with labor will allow you to explore many types of coping methods. Then you can think about what methods you may want to try in labor.

During your labor, when you feel the urge to push, you'll understand what the word *pressure* really means. Having gentle guidance and loving support is vital as you work hard to welcome your baby. The birth team will help ease your newborn into your waiting arms. They'll help you to bond, to fall in love with your baby, and become a mother. You'll feel ready to mother because you've already become a good parent by first becoming a good consumer of healthcare. The process of learning, asking, sharing, communicating and cooperating usually leads to good and safe decisions.

What if you have a cesarean birth? Making informed choices will lead to greater satisfaction, regardless of how your baby enters the world. Understanding ways to avoid a cesarean will affect your decision-making and will certainly influence the outcome of your birth. And your birth team's reactions and responses will have an impact on you, especially when an unexpected situation arises. Think carefully about whom you'll want at your birth.

Bonding and the first nursing are two of the most special events in your life as a new mother. Spending time with your baby and learning about newborn care will be your focus. Having a continuing thread of support from your human environment will help you have greater success and a smoother transition into mothering. So let people help you!

Since fatigue is the real enemy during the postpartum period, support from others continues to be critical. Your food, clothing, and shelter should be a loved one's responsibility. Your job is to get to know your child and continue falling in love—"babymooning," as it is sometimes called. Again, let people help!

Becoming a new mom is a *commencement*—the beginning of a new phase of life. It's when you graduate from adulthood into parenthood. Like any graduation, mixed feelings are normal. You will be excited about the baby, but you may also feel a loss of your past life when you had fewer responsibilities. This is similar to feelings you probably experienced when you graduated from school and had newfound responsibilities.

"Commencement" is a good term because it means the ending of one phase of your life to make way for a new, more challenging phase of your life. It is a beginning. Giving birth is not just a way to expand your family—it's your graduation toward a new life of parenting. Enjoy!

With time, your need for support will grow and change. Breastfeeding and parenting groups provide wonderful ways to meet other parents with common interests and concerns. Many lasting friendships develop from women striking up a conversation at a La Leche League meeting, for example.

When it comes to birth and parenting, there's a lot to consider. But it's not overwhelming. Most of it should just feel right to you. Don't overthink it, and don't look for problems. Have faith in yourself, in the process, and in the human environment you choose to support you. As a parent, you'll learn to go with your gut, and birth is a testing ground of sorts. Get excited, let others share in your excitement, and stay excited all the way along your journey to becoming a mother. Greet this rite of passage with all the wisdom, power, and resources you have.

Chapter 2
The Five Arms of Doula Support

One morning, a mother and daughter went for a walk along the ocean's edge. They came upon a stretch of beach that was littered with starfish, all washed ashore after a storm at sea the night before.

The little girl started picking them up and throwing them back into the water. Her mother told her to stop wasting her time—it would be impossible to save them all.

"Maybe I can't save them all," the little girl said, "but at least I can save one at a time."

Doulas are Like the Daughter

That's just the way doulas feel about the women they help. It's not that women need saving quite the same way the starfish did. But doulas feel the need to help them avoid problems that can occur before, during, and after the birth. Since this is such a special event in the woman's life, the doula is there to preserve and foster the mother's philosophy, preferences, and priorities—the things the mother has outlined in her birth vision.

By giving her the support she needs, the doula helps the mother prepare for, deal with, and recover from the birth better than she would have been able to do without help. The whole experience is safer, more successful, and more satisfying for mother, baby, partner, and family. Everybody wins.

We think of doula support as having five arms—just like a starfish:

1. *Spiritual.* A doula is a nurturing connection: she respects and honors the mutual womanhood she shares with the mother.

2. *Mediatorial.* A doula is a caring protector, representing the mother and helping her reach the goals in her personal birth vision through mediation.

3. *Physical.* A doula is a woman's personal handmaiden. She provides just about any personal comfort measure that the woman requests.

4. *Emotional.* A doula is the mother's trusted friend. She offers the mother encouragement and reassurance to soothe her mind.

5. *Informational.* A doula is a reliable resource. She feeds the mother's intellect, so she can make good decisions and feel empowered.

Spiritual Support

Although spiritual support can take the form of religion (if all are comfortable with that), it can also mean a *woman-to-woman connection*. Many cultures still provide special care and treatment for expectant or new mothers by other women. That's the doula concept in action! A lot of families in the United States lack that nurturing support system that can be provided by others—such as friends, neighbors, religious associates, or professionals like doulas.

Penny Simkin, one of the founders of DONA, did a study where she asked women about their birth experiences 25 years afterwards. What she determined was that giving birth is "not just another day in a woman's life."

Childbearing is not simply a means to expand your family. It is a rite of passage that will help define who this new woman is after meeting the challenges of birth. It is a unique opportunity for you to dig deep to discover your inner wisdom and strengths. If you listen to your body, you'll use its natural resources to develop self-coping techniques. These innate responses will combine to help you find your *inner birth vision* if you listen (and if others don't interfere with those messages). You can also benefit from wisdom through the ages, as the woman-to-woman connection blossoms in that birth space. The sympathy and empathy displayed towards you while you're in labor (by the doula, for instance) will encourage you, reassure you, guide you, and help you through this incredible task.

Some women find it difficult to surrender to others and actually let them help. You might be so used to handling things on your own that it may seem odd or uncomfortable to put trust in another when you're feeling so vulnerable. It may be because of something like personality type, career choice, upbringing, or even abuse. This is why developing a touch-and-trust relationship with your support team before the birth is important. Doulas spend a lot of time cultivating that kind of rapport with their client, so their woman-to-woman connection will develop. Without honest communication and unconditional trust, you can fall off the path on your journey to becoming a confident mother. Spiritual support on whatever level you prefer will offer you the additional strength and will to go forward.

Praying, chanting, singing hymns, etc. are also a beautiful way to include your religion in the birth, because they are effective on several levels. Religion itself brings comfort to all who believe. Emotional comfort leads to confidence and inner strength. Praying with others builds community and a sense of stability or connectedness. This can be your anchor in the choppy waters of labor. Verbal religious expressions are also often rhythmical in nature, which helps a woman cope. You might hold a rosary during labor if you're Catholic, for instance, and you and your doula might say "Hail Marys." Or you might have the family and the whole birth team hold hands to bless that baby and all who helped. Dad might sing hymns to the newborn while mommy is being taken care of, or you might have religious music to listen to during the birth and also during the bonding and nursing. A Buddhist might set up a small altar to chant to during labor. You might hold your beads and chant during each contraction. Whatever brings comfort to you in your cultural and religious traditions is also a good thing to share with the other people on your birth team. You'll probably find that they'll be fascinated by the opportunity to learn about traditions they've never encountered before.

It is important to make sure that everyone knows your cultural or religious preferences, traditions, or requests, so they can be respected. Many staff members or others outside of your family may not be accustomed to these beliefs or practices. Just a little education from the family helps your birth team proceed in a more sensitive manner. Any personal request usually has importance behind it, and it should be nurtured and protected by the birth team on your behalf.

The spiritual component of birth is certainly a powerful one and needs to be considered. To be able to tap into a personal belief that will bring you comfort and strength could well be the most critical area of your support. Don't be afraid to explore it, reveal it, and embrace it! After all, it's part of who you are. It will help mold you during that miraculous event we call birth.

Mediatorial Support

Advocate – a person who argues for a cause; a supporter or defender; a person who pleads on another's behalf; an intercessor.

Mediator – a person who resolves or settles differences by acting as an intermediary between parties; a person who intervenes to bring about an agreement, settlement, or compromise.

Advocacy is more confrontational; mediation is more cooperative.

When applying these two very different approaches to childbirth, timing is everything. During pregnancy, you should be your own advocate: investigate what your childbirth options are and communicate them to the doctor or midwife. Having a partner or doula to advocate more on your behalf can be a powerful addition. That's why we suggest that you and your partner attend as many appointments together as possible. It makes your mutual investment in this upcoming event evident to the whole birth team. There really is strength in numbers.

If you and your partner educate yourselves, ask questions about your caregiver's and hospital's policies, think about what options you'd like to try, and discuss them with your healthcare provider, you're setting yourselves up for success. You're taking responsibility for yourselves and making informed decisions. Since we know it can be unpredictable during the delivery, this sense of control *before* the birth can be very empowering. If you feel as though you've allowed others to control your birth because you're too passive in nature, you may have some emotional baggage to get over after the birth. Research has shown that pain and length of labor worry women the most before the birth. Afterwards, the things women regret the most are making poor choices and not participating enough.

We doulas like to talk about your "locus of control," which is one of the main things that affect how you view the outcome of your birth. Assertive women who determine their own fate through personal actions and take responsibility for the consequences of those decisions have an *internal* locus of control. Passive women who let others determine their fate through words and actions have an *external* locus of control. Many women feel swept away and crumble once they get to the birthplace, forgetting that they have a voice about what's happening. Even partners can succumb to the more medical practices associated with birthing today, especially if tired or overwhelmed emotionally. To prevent this from happening, investing in a birth vision and using mediation during your birth is critical. You learn to be a good consumer, which is a lifelong asset—especially for a new parent.

Several decades ago, the term *family-centered maternity care* was introduced. It shifted the focus off the medical practitioner's or the hospital's policy and onto the patient and her family, where it belongs. Physiologic childbirth, birth plans, rooming-in, communicating with doctors, and staff cooperation evolved from this movement to create a more family-based model in obstetrics. The mother and her wishes were to be paramount over common procedures and standard protocol. Routine use of interventions decreased...for a while. Then, with what we call the epidural epidemic in the 90's, interventions to monitor and maintain the regional anesthesia became more common. Many hospitals started to assume that all women wanted or needed epidurals, and routine interventions crept back into American childbirth.

What happened in the last 50 years that made women feel they can't birth without drugs or interventions? For hundreds of thousands of years, women used their natural resources and social support. Let's bring back what worked! Women listening to their bodies, so they can find their birth rhythm—that should be everyone's goal. And we can reach that goal with an appropriate mix of advocacy and mediation.

Use mediation during your birth to make it a more positive experience. If your doctor or midwife has a different sense of how things should go during your birth, asking for time to discuss it is very helpful. You can gather information about your options from your doula (or staff) to make an informed decision upon their return. Using open-ended questions is always useful, since it results in open dialogue, instead of getting yes or no answers. So begin questions with *who, what, when, where, why*, or *how*.

"Active listening" can help you figure out what someone is trying to convey. Begin the sentence with; "It sounds like..." and add to it what you think they are trying to say. What you heard may not be what they intended to communicate at all. Summarizing the end result of the conversation is also very important. It focuses on what the team decided after discussing all options and leaves no room for confusion. After all, you and your partner are adults utilizing a service. So, wherever possible, your feelings, needs, and choices should be listened to and respected by those attending you.

A Common Scenario

No mediation:

Resident (after an exam) – It's time to break your water.

Mom – What?

Resident – You're not dilating a centimeter per hour. In fact, you're still three centimeters.

Partner – We don't want to do that.

Resident – I think we should, to speed things up...so she doesn't get tired. What if she can't push and needs a cesarean?

Mom or partner – Oh, then we'd better do it.

With mediation:

Resident (after an exam) – It's time to break your water.

Mom – What?

Resident – You're not dilating a centimeter per hour. In fact, you're still three centimeters.

Doula – It sounds like you're not pleased with the dilation.

Resident – Well, she could get tired at this rate.

Doula – What other progress has she made beyond dilation?

Resident – She's effaced a bit more.

Partner – Well, that is progress, isn't it?

Resident – Yes, but not much.

Doula – What is the effacement now?

Resident – One hundred per cent.

Doula – And what is the baby's station?

Resident – He's come down from minus one to zero station.

Doula – Wow! Those are two good changes. Now we have to work on helping that cervix to dilate.

Resident – We can use pitocin for that.

Mom – I'm afraid it will hurt more with the water gone and pitocin.

Resident – That's what epidurals are for.

Partner – What? How did we get to epidurals?

Doula – How do you feel about us trying some specific things, like squatting or showering, to help with progress before breaking her water?

Resident – Well, rupturing the membrane and pitocin works the best.

Doula – What would you say to giving us an hour, so we can do these techniques that the couple was hoping to try first before using interventions?

Resident – Well, since the baby is okay, we can wait a while. I'll check back in an hour.

Partner– Oh good.

Doula – Thank you, Doctor, we appreciate your cooperation. We'll see you in an hour to discuss our options then.

Resident – OK.

Having a caring protector in the room, such as a doula, will reassure you and your partner in many ways. Her caring detachment enables her to represent you calmly, to ask questions on your behalf, to request time for you to determine your choice, and to intervene when you may feel unable to handle the situation. Her knowledge and expertise can provide you with information, guidance, and support that many women and their partners find extremely valuable.

How you express your preferences is critical. You can be assertive without being aggressive. Being aggressive is a technique more aligned with advocacy. To argue or plead does not usually end with a favorable result. Mediating, on the other hand, generally results in arriving at decisions that everyone can live with. Doulas learn these skills in training and use them in non-offensive ways at many appointments or births they attend. Doulas are there to nurture and protect the mother's birth experience. They represent the mother while maintaining professional decorum to help create a positive and lasting memory for the woman and her family.

Being proactive in this regard really pays off. Bringing caring and creative members to the birth team will make the human environment more supportive and give you more emotional stamina. A birth vision that reflects your philosophy, preferences, and priorities will guide the birth team, so they can help you accomplish what is important to you and avoid what you most want to avoid. Although the staff should not force their personal birth philosophy on you, some do. This can lead to decision-making based on their agenda, not yours. And that can contribute to your feeling regret or remorse afterwards. This is why a written birth vision is so important—it protects everyone and encourages all to maintain their place within the birth team. This truly is your own personal right of passage.

Physical Support

Physical support is anything that helps you feel as comfortable as possible and well taken care of. A birth doula, for instance, considers herself to be the mother's personal handmaiden, helping with everything from massages to bathroom breaks. The right physical support at the right time can help you deal with pain without drugs and can help your labor progress better.

Movements and position changes are one important aspect of physical support. Every mother and every birth is unique; the same position isn't best for everyone. Even when you find the position that seems most comfortable to you, changing positions every once in a while is still a good idea. Labor usually makes better progress when you can move. Rhythmical movements can help you cope with pain.

There are plenty of techniques that can help with different parts of labor or with different kinds of pain. A good doula knows many different things to try, and it's always helpful to have thought a little in advance about which ones you might like to use during your labor.

Massage is another good way of coping with pain and relaxing, so your body can do its work. Just the touch of someone you trust is comforting. The right kind of touch can actually reduce the pain you feel.

Hydrotherapy—like taking a bath—makes labor easier and faster for many women, so can the right application of heat or cold at the right time.

You'll also want to think about food and drink. Your midwife or doctor will tell you what the rules are, but it's important that you get at least some nutrition and hydration, so that you'll have enough energy to meet the physical challenges of labor.

A birth ball can help with movements you might want to try during labor. There are a lot of other tools you might want, too: hot water bottle, cold compresses, massage oil, and so on. You'll want to make a list of things you'll need and have your birth bag packed and ready to go well ahead of time. (Check out our suggestions for what to include in Chapter 4 and how to cope using ideas in Chapters 5 and 6.)

Emotional Support

The need for emotional support varies greatly from one mom to the next. All women need this kind of support, but to different degrees, at different times, and from different people.

If it's your first birth, fear of the unknown can be a real roadblock in labor. Your support team should be prepared for this and have strategies in place to guide you, keep you informed, and include you in decision making.

If you've had a previous traumatic birth experience, your greatest emotional challenge may be how to prevent similar circumstances from happening again. The human environment you've chosen needs to help you by being more proactive than last time, by pointing out differences from before, and by maintaining a positive attitude that will become contagious for you.

If you're a single mom, family and staff will have to support your emotional needs, since a significant other may not be in the picture. Getting to know your birth team before the birth helps you build the trust you'll need to rely on during the birth.

Trust, locus of control, and privacy all figure into the emotional-support equation. Trust during a vulnerable time is hard for a woman, particularly when pain, tension, and fatigue cloud her mind. The birth team needs to spearhead that effort, so you can ease into feeling comfortable with your surroundings—human and inanimate. You need a birth team that can help you set up your nest, feel free to labor, and find your birth groove. If you have the encouragement and reassurance of those surrounding you, you'll feel empowered and capable of doing this job. *You are not alone*...these are powerful words.

Your locus of control determines whether you are assertive or passive in nature. An assertive individual has an internal locus of control: you determine your own destiny through personal decision-making. If you have an external locus of control, you give that control over to others who influence your fate. Many women approach birth very passively, especially if it's their first baby. Fear of the unknown, lack of confidence in their bodies, poor education, and controlling healthcare providers are some of the reasons for women feeling that way. You can gain mastery if you have the opportunity to learn, have the right attitude, and go in prepared with appropriate skills.

Privacy is an important factor to consider during the birth. You deserve the right to labor as you choose, with all those in attendance respectful of your needs. Keeping the door shut, putting a *please knock* sign on the door, keeping the curtain drawn, and always making sure anyone attending you identifies themselves to you are some important considerations. If your vulnerability is lessened through these simple steps, that's a way of further protecting your emotional well-being.

Difficult situations like a prolonged early phase of labor, very long births, and some medical outcomes can be emotionally stressful for a laboring woman. A woman who goes into labor after days of unproductive contractions may already feel defeated. If she feels totally exhausted, all her emotions can get blurred. A birth filled with medical interventions can be traumatic for someone who expected a more normal and natural one. All that fear and despair can keep the mother from moving forward in her birth—and it's hard on family members, too. But it's important to recognize and deal with those emotions. Someone with a caring detachment, like a doula, won't get swept away as other loved ones might.

The unexpected can dramatically influence how a woman handles a birth emotionally. If the baby has an anomaly, is a stillbirth, or requires intensive care, the woman clearly will be devastated. Still, she needs to birth the baby and mother it to whatever extent is possible. This is so hard when her heart is breaking! Those around her can try to be mindful of her pain and respectful of her need to release it. Allowing her to express her feelings with complete freedom will help her on her way through the grieving process. Any time there is a loss, grief must follow for healing to happen. A professional, like a doula, is trained in skills to help the mother explore her grief and work through the feelings of loss.

New roles and the adjustment to these new roles begin at birth for the parents. You'll be recovering from the birth, and you'll certainly have fatigue, doubts, and lack of confidence to deal with. The family can easily feel overwhelmed. Preparing for the difficult times associated with postpartum will often prevent them from happening. Simple reminders like eating properly, sleeping often, limiting visitors, and prioritizing chores can turn an insane household into a more manageable one. If someone offers help afterwards, take it. For example, enjoy their casserole, give them a shopping list, have them do a small load of wash, and take them up on the chance to sleep while they watch the baby. Accepting help and dividing the jobs up can accomplish a lot, while you recover and fall in love with your new baby.

Postpartum mood disorders (anything from "baby blues" to psychosis) can be lessened with support at the birth. When a woman feels empowered by her birth experience, she shows it…in a positive way. When a woman is belittled by her birth experience, she also shows it…often in a negative way. It can show up as depression—and that can really affect how she mothers. It is critical for those around her to be on the lookout for signs, so action can be taken. It may mean more sleep, paid help, ordering food out, support groups, or that counseling is indicated. The responsibility of a newborn is pretty overwhelming for new moms without the added burden of depression. This is why generations of new mothers counted on help and guidance from other experienced women to assist with their transition into parenthood. Unfortunately, that kind of support is often lacking within modern-day families. Enter the postpartum doula!

The postpartum doula picks up where the birth doula leaves off. She goes to the home, provides family care, does light housekeeping, prepares meals, and runs short errands to keep the household running smoothly. She helps the family learn about breastfeeding, infant care, time management, organizational skills, and so on. She gently guides them into feeling confident about their new role as parents.

And the doula is also there to pick up on any concerns that may interfere with the family's success. This can be very reassuring to the new parents, who are probably feeling just plain overworked by this little bundle of joy.

Emotions are part of what separate us from the animals when giving birth. Animals just do their instinctive thing. We humans let emotions get in our way through many of life's events. Becoming a mother is definitely one of the most emotional events in a woman's life. Recognizing that and preparing for it will set her up for greater success.

Informational Support

Every woman wants to know what her labor will feel like and be like. Most women who are supported in their birth choices can have a satisfying birth. Many women are amazed to find how well they were able to cope with their labor.

Having reliable information makes a big difference on the outcome of your birth. Knowing what your choices are and making your own decisions will go a long way toward making your birth an empowering rite of passage. A doula can be a reliable resource of information to help you make informed choices about your birth. You and your doula can have a series of dialogues before your birth. In these conversations, she presents the best information she has regarding local birth practices and current national research, and discusses your preferences in light of the information.

How does good information affect the outcome of your birth experience? If birth is a natural physiologic process that any dolphin knows how to do without childbirth classes, why should you worry about being so informed? The difference is, we live in a medicalized society. Women who are not well informed are much *less* likely to have a more natural childbirth. If you don't know what your choices are, you can easily lose control. You're more likely to have medical interventions, and you're less likely to know why you're having them. Most hospitals and surgeons have routine procedures that make it much more likely that your birth experience will be managed as a medical event—unless you know enough to make your own informed decisions.

Birth is cultural, the way eating is cultural. We don't just eat what our bodies need to sustain us. If we only did that, there would be no reason for birthday cake. Birthday cake is part of our food culture. The place you are giving birth in has a local culture as well. It also partakes of our national birth culture. Not everything doctors do regarding birth makes the birth faster or physically easier for you or the baby. Some things are just cultural. For example, most hospitals do not offer enemas to birthing women anymore, yet a few years ago, most women who labored in hospitals were required to have an enema, whether they wanted one or not. Enemas are sometimes helpful at birth, but not always. They don't usually affect the medical outcome much. But they used to be part of the birthing culture. We have a local hospital that gives new families who want one a candlelight champagne dinner for the three of them the day after their baby's birth. It isn't necessary for postpartum care, but isn't it nice?

Only you can decide whether an obstetrician, a family-practice doctor, or a midwife is right for your birth. But without good information to help you make your choice, you might be swept along with the tide of medical procedures—procedures that might make your birth a less comfortable and a less positive experience for you. The less you know about your birthing options, the more likely you will have interventions that are unnecessary for you. How will you know if they are necessary or not? You don't need to become a doctor—you just need to become an informed consumer of healthcare.

When you have the five arms of doula support in place, you'll be able to have a successful and satisfying birth. You'll be certain that your birth team will know and respect your wishes. You'll be well informed and be able to make the right choices for you—choices which you won't have to worry about and regret later.

All that is true, whether you have a professional doula with you or not. Naturally, we think it's always best to have a doula. But you need to have that support somehow—whether it's from a doula, family members, or friends. If you have the right support, you can relax and allow your body to birth the way it was meant to.

Chapter 3

Envisioning Your Birth

The bride was looking forward to her big day. She and her fiancé had planned all the details. She had chosen her favorite flowers to carry, roses and orchids. They had chosen the wedding music together, as well as the song for their first dance at the reception: "It Had to Be You." She had selected a wonderful dress to wear made of silk and lace. They had invited their closest friends and relatives to participate with them in the ceremony. They had planned the ceremony together down to the smallest detail. The invitations had been sent, and their family and friends were going to witness their union.

She had literally spent months planning each detail of the ceremony and the reception party afterwards. She knew what her wedding cake would taste like and how it would look. She had chosen a luscious variety of foods for her guests to eat. She was going to be a princess for a day.

As her wedding day dawned, she carefully dressed herself, her friends assisting her. She looked her most beautiful. She walked down the aisle, feeling a bit nervous. The ceremony seemed like something out of a dream. Afterwards, at the reception, she was delighted that her friends and family were enjoying themselves. She and her brand new spouse were celebrating their special day to remember.

Envisioning Your Big Day

Most women plan their weddings very carefully. You've probably dreamed about the details for a long time—dreamed about everything from how you would look to how happy you would be when you exchanged vows. You realize that a wedding takes a lot of planning. You want the day to be joyful for you and all your family and friends, so you add your own special touches to make the day uniquely yours.

All that planning takes a lot of time and emotional energy. But that investment pays off in the satisfaction you feel as you enjoy the wedding—and pays off even more in the happy memories years afterward.

But how many women spend as much time thinking about the birth of a child as they do about a wedding? Just like a wedding day, the birth day of your child is a very significant occasion. It is a day you will always remember.

Penny Simkin, one of the founders of Doulas of North America, asked women 25 years after their birth experiences what it meant to them. What her research showed was that birth is "not just another day in a woman's life." The research showed that the moms remembered more negative feelings than positive ones. Many of the women remembered the way the staff treated them—whether it was positive or negative. The human environment is very important. The day you give birth will matter to you forever.

There are some elements that are similar in every wedding, as well as those touches a woman adds to make hers unique. The same is true of birth. Birth is universal and has elements that every woman experiences. But if we spent just a fraction of the time thinking about a birth that we spend on planning a wedding, we'd be well prepared. A mother-to-be would be able to add the special touches that would comfort her and help her *celebrate* the day, not just get through it.

That's why we think every mother-to-be should have a *birth vision.*

We like to say "birth vision" rather than "birth plan." Birth is a natural process, and nature is in command. You can never *plan* exactly what will happen. But *envisioning* your birth, rather than *planning* it, will empower you, yet not set you up for failing to meet your expectations. Following a birth vision rather than a detailed birth plan gives you flexibility during birth. Being open-minded is important, but so is having goals. You want to be proactive, not reactive. Thinking about issues before they happen helps you handle them better if they do happen. Reacting to an unexpected situation is much harder during a contraction or after many hours of labor.

A birth vision is a couple's blending of philosophies, preferences, and priorities. It helps foster good communication, respect, and cooperation throughout the birth team. Everyone knows in advance what you want, and you have the confidence of knowing that you're an educated consumer.

Being an Educated Consumer

We don't often think of ourselves as healthcare *consumers,* but we ought to think that way. We have choices to make, options to consider, and personal preferences to figure out. We should be at least as picky in our healthcare as we are when we're making wedding plans.

Being a good consumer means educating yourself, preparing in advance, and making informed decisions. It's work. But the rewards are great. When you have a process to follow, you'll make better choices, and you'll have few—if any—regrets. You won't have to deal with the emotional baggage many women carry after their births because they made uninformed decisions during the birth.

It's also better for everyone else on your birth team—doctor, midwife, nurse, doula, partner, or anyone else in the room. If you've made your choices in advance, then everyone already knows what you want. Everyone has a better sense of control and participation. No one has to guess what you want.

It's Your Vision

The only agenda that's important at a birth is the mother's. The whole human environment should strive to be respectful and supportive of this critical component. You, the mother, should choose how to birth and parent and protect and nurture—not anyone else. If a user-friendly birth vision is available to healthcare providers, you can form a working alliance with them to meet your own wants and needs better. There's no us-versus-them: everyone is working for the same objective. And no personal or professional agendas can override yours when your birth vision is honored. The birth remains more woman-centered, instead of becoming medically oriented.

A birth vision gives you and your partner a chance to discover and verbalize your personal feelings, concerns, and goals, and then incorporate them into the birth journey. You should discuss all your feelings and ideas about birth, so you and your partner, and the entire birth team, can respect them when it's time to meet the baby.

There's another reason why a birth vision is important: it helps shape the outcome for mom and baby. Not being involved in your own care can result in your turning into a patient, rather than being a laboring woman. Then you can end up having intervention after intervention, like dominoes falling one after another.

Losing control that way can have negative effects on both you and your baby—short-term and long-term. Your own physical recovery can take longer, and you may have more trouble adjusting emotionally to postpartum life. And interventions can adversely affect your baby's health and relationship to you.

Birth is a physiological event, not a pathological one. If you follow your own body's messages and draw on its natural resources, you'll find your birth groove and inherent rhythm. If you let others direct you and make the decisions for you, they've taken away your opportunity to experience the rite of passage in becoming a mother. And how you feel about that will help shape you as you transition into parenthood.

The sooner you start thinking specifically about *your* birth the better chance you have to make your birth vision come true, or as close to true as you can. While you are thinking through the possibilities of what might happen during birth, you will ask your caregivers what their protocols are. You can discover if there are incompatibilities between you and your caregivers' procedures. You will start to explore what will be the most comfortable for you during birth. You will figure out how to get the things in your birth that are the most important to you.

Building Relationships

Scenario One - She arrived for her appointment and checked in with the receptionist. They called her back to do her blood pressure, weight check, and urine test. She continued into the exam room and waited until the healthcare provider arrived. He asked how she was doing, measured her fundal height, and did the internal exam. He told her there was nothing happening and proceeded to do the beta strep culture. He then told her to make another appointment a week from now and left. She got dressed, made another appointment, and went back to work.

This is what is often called an uneventful appointment because nothing out of the ordinary happened. In reality, it was uneventful...period! There was no meaningful dialogue between mother and doctor; questions weren't asked, issues weren't discussed, and no real rapport was established. Rewind and try again.

Scenario Two - She arrived for her appointment and checked in with the receptionist. They called her back to do her blood pressure, weight check, and urine test. She pulled out her pregnancy journal and marked down all the information, so she could report the details back to her partner. She asked the nurse how on time the doctor was running and what was planned that day during the appointment.

The nurse mentioned the beta strep test and the mom asked what it was, how it was done, and what her alternatives were if she was positive. The nurse pulled out a pamphlet describing the culture and left it with the mom while she waited for the doctor.

When the doctor arrived, he asked how she was doing. She gave him a report and asked about the beta strep test. He explained it briefly and told her he'd do an exam and then the test. She asked if she could do the test herself, and he agreed to give her the instructions.

Next the doctor examined her internally and announced that nothing was happening. She asked specific questions about the direction of the cervix, effacement, dilation, baby's station and position.

The doctor was impressed by her questions and asked how she knew so much about pregnancy. She told him about the classes she'd taken and the books she was reading. She mentioned that she and her partner were working on their written birth vision and had hired a doula for the birth. He expressed interest in meeting the doula and seeing the birth vision. He told her to make an appointment for next week, reminded her when to call if she thought she was in labor, and told her to ask about the test results next time.

She jotted down a summary of their discussion and got dressed. She went into the restroom to do the culture and then made her appointment for the next week. She went back to work and called her partner about the great appointment she'd had with the doctor that day.

What a difference between scenario one and two! Building relationships before the birth is a critical piece of developing the human environment that's right for you. Feeling confident in your care, feeling well informed, feeling reassured by your support, and feeling that others truly respect your choices–all these things empower you. They give you the sense that the birth task ahead of you is achievable—with help!

Relationships with healthcare providers, staff, educators, doulas, family, and friends influence how you will respond to the birth. If you have a passive attitude, you'll let others influence you and make decisions for you. After the birth, you might end up feeling that you surrendered control to others. But if you're assertive, you'll accept the responsibility of your decisions and the consequences of your actions. What you put into it, you get out of it.

The Winning Combination

You can see now how much of an effect education, preparation, and attitude have on the birth outcome. Take control of what you can control. Preparation through learning and practicing—physical and mental conditioning—will improve your chances of tolerating the pain and length of labor. Knowing what to expect and what to do is the answer.

It all comes down to embracing childbirth as physiological, not pathological. That's the winning attitude. The two birthing philosophies are compared in Table 1.

Table 1. Physiologic Birth versus Medical Birth

Physiologic Birth	Medical Birth
Normal, healthy activity	Potentially hazardous event
Watchful waiting approach	Time constraints imposed
Self-regulatory behavior	Control by staff
Others listen & cooperate	Others inform & direct
Mother provides valuable cues	Data from interventions rule
Touch is for support & pain relief	Touch is procedural
Interventions only if necessary	Interventions used routinely
Family-centered maternity care*	Medically oriented maternity care

*What is family-centered maternity care? Just what its name implies—care that reflects what is important to the family, not what is routine or convenient for the staff. Family-centered maternity care focuses on listening to the family's philosophy, respecting their preferences and being mindful of their priorities. It's treating the woman and her significant others in such a way that this birth day truly is a special birthday.

Natural Birth versus Birthing *Naturally*

What does "natural childbirth" mean? Some think natural childbirth means a vaginal birth. To others, it means no drugs were used. And to others, it means squatting in a rice paddy to birth (and then going back to work!).

So let's forget about "natural childbirth." The words mean too many things to too many people. Instead, we'll switch the words around and talk about *birthing naturally*.

Birthing naturally means following your own body's instincts—letting your body do the job it was designed to do. Beyond that, of course, it can mean whatever you want it to mean. That's the beauty of having choices. Just remember that your own body gives you a lot of natural resources to draw on:

- *Listen to your body.* Your body was made to do this job. Be confident in it! Remember that your anatomy and physiology is wonderfully designed to make, carry, and birth a baby. Your body will send you messages—you just need to be open to hearing them. Listening to your gut really applies in this case.

- *Endorphins.* Your body releases special hormones, called *endorphins,* to combat the pain of birth. By keeping you as relaxed as possible, your team can reduce the amount of adrenalin that may also be released in labor (through fear or anxiety), which cancels out your endorphins. So try to enjoy relaxation by communicating and cooperating with your birth team throughout labor.

- *Natural pain relief.* You may find that pressure on certain points in your body makes contractions pick up, but feel less painful (see chapter 5). So be open to different methods of pain relief!

- *Lips, feet, hands.* When your lips, the soles of your feet, and the palms of your hands are stimulated during labor, you feel less pain. So lick your lips often and squeeze stress balls during contractions!

- *Massage.* Get a hand massage or soak your feet in scented water while laboring—you'll release endorphins and feel less pain.

- *Gate control.* Your body's largest organ is the skin. Its nerve endings are very close to the surface, so we sense hot, cold, sharp, etc. instantaneously. This contributes to our safety and survival as humans. If the skin is stimulated by touch, massage, pressure, vibration, warmth, cold, or water during labor, you will feel less pain from the contraction. The *gate control theory* kicks in and reduces the amount of pain you feel from the contraction traveling along deeper nerve pathways to get to the brain. After receiving messages from the skin, the brain begins assimilating those stimuli. So by the time the contraction pain arrives, the brain is busy; a gate drops, and less pain gets in. So get in the Jacuzzi during the most intense part of labor!

Natural Flow

Have you ever noticed that all of nature is repetitive? The pattern of the waves, the cycles of the moon, the changing of the seasons, the mating behaviors of animals—just to name a few. So why not use rhythm to enhance your own birth? If you allow yourself the freedom to find your birth groove, your natural flow will take over. That means you need to be a woman, not a lady, to give birth.

If you want to moan or grunt or verbalize rhythmically during a contraction, it often helps. So don't worry about how you sound—just express yourself however you need to. You might find listening to music or repetitive sounds to be helpful, too.

Movement can also add to the rhythmical nature of birth. March in place, wiggle your hips, or sway your body during contractions. These are normal ways of *self-soothing*. Rocking back and forth when experiencing gas pains, for example, seems to be a natural response, because it's soothing and repetitive. Swaying back and forth can calm a fussy baby because it's soothing and rhythmical. Get the idea?

Natural Comforts

What brings you comfort? Is it a beautiful sunset? Your grandmother's chicken noodle soup? Being wrapped in a down blanket? Think about what might bring comfort to you while in labor: a favorite stuffed animal, a certain kind of music, soft candlelight, a good book, the smell of bread baking, a fluffy pillow, or warm chocolate-chip cookies. Use your five senses to consider what would make you feel more comfortable. Then you'll be more relaxed, less worried about the pain, and more confident in the process. You want to make the birth space yours—more homey and safe. Answer these quick birth questions to help you start thinking about your birth vision.

Ten Quick Birth Questions

1. What helps you to relax?
2. What has helped you deal with pain in the past?
3. What is your greatest concern regarding this birth?
4. What special requests might you have (personal, religious, cultural)?
5. What are you hoping to accomplish?
6. What are you hoping to avoid?
7. How are you hoping to be treated?
8. How do you envision the perfect space and place for birthing?
9. Who do you want to be there and why?
10. What would be YOUR ideal outcome?

Natural Methods

Finding the combination that works best for you is the key. Think about what combination of natural resources, natural flow, and natural comforts will help *you* in birthing naturally. That will be *your* personal method. To start developing your natural methods, try this birth art activity.

Birth Art Activity

1. Get a blank piece of paper and crayons.
2. Start creating what you'd want your birth space to be like and what natural comforts you'd want to include.
3. Use lots of color, texture, and imagination.
4. Then, draw yourself in it doing something you really want to try in labor. Yes you can use stick figures!

Table 2. Birth Your Way versus Birth Their Way

	Your way	*Their way*
Movement	You move as you wish.	You're kept in bed and monitored.
Timing	You're not timed; the process follows your body.	Your cervix is expected to dilate 1 centimeter per hour.
Pushing	You push in whatever position feels best.	You push in the position the staff tells you to push in.
Breastfeeding	Your baby nurses within the first half hour.	You can't hold your baby until after perineal repair.
Bonding	You hold your baby from the beginning.	The baby stays in the warmer; you don't hold your baby in the first hour.

Being a Savvy Consumer

If you're encouraged to believe in your innate ability to give birth, you'll meet the challenge. But if you're led down the path of doubting your ability and mistrusting your body, how can you succeed? It is the responsibility of your birth team to put your wants, needs, and decisions before anybody else's. So your partner and doula can influence staff in a positive way by demonstrating how you deserve to be treated.

Recognizing that the birth team members have different roles is also important. The care provider and staff are there mainly for medical care and attention. The partner and doula are there specifically for labor support. Family and friends might be there for social or moral support. Anyone who is not contributing to the overall effectiveness of the working alliance should be eliminated from the birth team. Only positive and constructive assistance is helpful. Negative words, tones, actions, and body language can greatly impact how you will handle the anxiety, pain, and fatigue associated with labor.

The more you learn about your choices in childbirth and the more you decide what is right for you, the more satisfying your relationship with your doctor or midwife will be. You need to be a savvy consumer of childbirth care, so that you can be secure in your decisions.

If you were having your car repaired, you might not have the technical expertise to repair the car yourself, but you would want to ask questions and be satisfied with your mechanic's answers. Your healthcare providers are just the same. They have expertise about childbirth, which is why you are hiring them to assist you. But you still need to be able to communicate your wishes and needs to them—or go elsewhere for care.

If you're expecting your first child, it can be difficult to be assertive. You're naturally concerned for your baby's health, and you're looking to experts to help you safeguard it. You may find it hard to start a useful dialogue with your care provider.

If your care provider is telling you something unexpected or something you did not already know, listen carefully. Try not to allow your fears to color what you hear. It often helps to take your partner or doula with you to an appointment. What they hear will probably be less worrisome than what you thought you heard. After listening, repeat back the information to be sure you heard it correctly. Listen, listen, listen.

Here are some tips for building your communication skills:

- Keep a list of questions, so you don't forget important personal issues.

- Give your list to the nurse just before the appointment begins to attach to your chart, or mention to the healthcare provider when she first arrives in the exam room that you have some issues to discuss.

- Use open-ended questions to avoid getting a yes or no answer and to stimulate dialogue. Begin your question with *who, what, when, where, why* or *how*…not *should, could, would, do, does,* and so on. Review important points before moving onto the next topic—so that you are clear about the response.

- Watch your tone of voice and attitude. Be assertive, not aggressive.

- Negotiate a compromise whenever it is needed. For example, ask for telemetric monitoring during labor if constant monitoring is required: that way you can still be mobile. (Telemetric monitors transmit their information wirelessly, so you don't have to be tied down to one spot.)

- Take your birth vision to an appointment. A copy can be placed in your file for other associates to see and comment upon. Give one to your doula, too, and take it to the birthplace with you.

- If you get an unacceptable answer or attitude about your birth vision or other requests, make another appointment to discuss it again. This time bring some support along (like your partner or doula). Or talk to another healthcare provider about the resistance you got from their associate.

- Find out if you need written orders from your doctor or midwife for any of your requests—for example, using the shower or Jacuzzi or having clear fluids and light food, in addition to ice chips in labor.

- If you have done your best and you are not satisfied with your caregiver, think about finding a caregiver you *will* be comfortable with.

Changing Your Mind

It's never too early in your pregnancy to start talking to your caregiver about your birth vision. You might have continued seeing the same physician who has been giving you routine pap smears for years. He may have been great for gynecological care, but you might discover that your priorities about birth are different from his. The earlier you find that out, the easier it will be for you to transfer your care to a more like-minded practitioner. There are five very important questions for you to answer about your caregiver:

1. How open is your care provider to having intelligent discussions with you? Without the give and take of dialogue before labor begins, how can you feel confident that your requests will be listened to during the far more vulnerable time of birth?

2. What is your caregiver's unmedicated birth rate? If his clients have a high epidural rate, he might be used to laboring mothers not changing positions, and he might not know how to deal with the more natural coping methods you're exploring.

3. What is your caregiver's rate of inductions? If his rate is high, it might mean that he is less patient with the birthing process. You'll also feel more pressured and worried if you go beyond your due date.

4. What is your caregiver's cesarean rate? The cesarean birthrate has skyrocketed in recent years. You want to feel confident that if you have a cesarean birth, it's because you really need one.

5. What is your caregiver's episiotomy rate? What is his instrument delivery rate (vacuum extraction or forceps delivery)? A discussion about episiotomies and instrument deliveries will tell you about your caregiver's attitude about a woman's body. Does he believe that a woman's body can usually give birth without intervention? Or does he feel that, most of the time, a woman's body needs medical assistance to give birth? Nearly everyone does some episiotomies and instrument deliveries, but you should know why and under what circumstances your caregiver does them.

Chapter 4

Getting Ready for the Birth

Body and Mind

Heather and Dror were naturally overjoyed to be expecting a child, and they planned everything to make the experience meaningful and memorable. Heather had Graves' Disease (an overactive thyroid), so she knew high-risk doctors would have to be involved in her care. But for the birth itself, she picked a male midwife with a first-rate reputation, and she had the best doula she knew. She and her husband went to all their childbirth classes together, and they took yoga together. Heather saw her chiropractor regularly, and she had pregnancy massages, as well. She planned to have a belly cast to commemorate her pregnancy. She expected to labor with no medications and as few interventions as possible. It would be a beautiful, natural, family-centered birth.

But things don't always go the way you plan. Almost 7 weeks before her due date, Heather was out shopping when she started feeling contractions. When she called her midwife, he told her to go home, relax, and see what happened. The contractions continued, so he advised her to go to the hospital. When they got there, Heather was told she was 2 centimeters dilated and becoming pre-eclamptic—which meant she would be staying until the baby was born. Immediately, she had to be given steroids to help mature the baby's lungs, drugs to stop contractions, and drugs to bring down her blood pressure. When the birth came, she and the baby would have to be monitored constantly, and she'd have a carousel of IV's and other interventions to deal with.

But Heather didn't give up on her idea of a family-centered birth. A few days later, the hospital allowed her doula to come in and make the belly cast Heather had always wanted. Later that evening, her water broke. Once the labor got going, the doctors and nurses were as quiet and unobtrusive as they could be, and her husband, midwife and doula helped Heather deliver in a lunge-squat position. She had no pain medication, and she didn't need an episiotomy. Less than 3 hours after her water broke, Heather welcomed baby Zeev into the world. He weighed 5½ pounds, and he adapted so well to his new environment that they were able to bond and try nursing before Zeev was taken to intensive care for observation—standard procedure for any baby who is 6 weeks early.

Between breastfeeding and kangaroo care (with both parents), Zeev thrived and was released in eight days. In spite of all the medical machinery, Heather still describes the birth as being very intimate and special. She appreciated that she was listened to and kept informed at all times, and that a medical birth could be managed in such a woman-centered way. Because she was determined to have a joyful birth and because she was ready to adapt when her circumstances changed, she was able to enjoy the meaningful and memorable experience she'd planned from the beginning. She had set herself up for success and achieved it—even when things didn't go quite the way she'd hoped.

A Grandmother Is Born

That's the story of the how Jan became a grandmother after having been a doula to other young mothers for over 30 years. (Yes, of course, Jan was the doula in the story.) Birth is always an amazing journey, but it may have unexpected twists and turns. Just remember that, wherever the path takes you, you can have a positive memory of your birth and a wonderful story to tell.

Helping Your Body Prepare

As the baby drops (called lightening), shortness of breath and indigestion disappear. But there are trade-offs. When the baby moves down in the last weeks, you might feel pressure on the bladder and lower back. Moms often feel like they have to run to the bathroom, only to find that their bladder wasn't nearly as full as it felt. To help reduce the risk of wetting your pants (especially when laughing, sneezing, or coughing), try doing the Kegel exercise.

This pelvic-floor-strengthening exercise not only reduces incontinence, but it also prepares your "bottom" for birth. By tightening and then relaxing the figure 8 of muscles that surround the vagina and rectum, you make the area healthier and better conditioned to do the work associated with birthing. Do Kegels several times a day in the weeks leading up to the birth. Many women connect doing Kegels to something they do frequently, like eating a meal or making a trip to the bathroom. Or you might put reminder notes around the house or in your date book.

To identify the pelvic floor muscles, stop the flow of urine *only once* while emptying your bladder. If you stop and start frequently while urinating, it could lead to incomplete emptying of the bladder and infection.

Here are two variations of the Kegel exercise that might help.

Super Kegels – Pull your pelvic floor muscles in and up and try to hold for a count of 20. If the muscles begin to drop, pull them back up until 20. Remember to keep breathing as you exercise.

Elevator Exercise – Sit comfortably in a chair with your feet flat on the ground. Pull your muscles up gradually like you're ascending in an elevator floor by floor. After reaching the 5th floor (Baby Department—what else?), slowly lower the muscles until you reach the ground floor (sitting on the chair). Now, press the muscles down against the chair as you bulge to the basement level. This will help you coordinate your efforts when you may feel confused as to how to direct your power when pushing the baby out. Kegels are also recommended to do after the birth to help with perineal and rectal healing. We've included an illustration of the woman's internal reproductive organs (Figure 1).

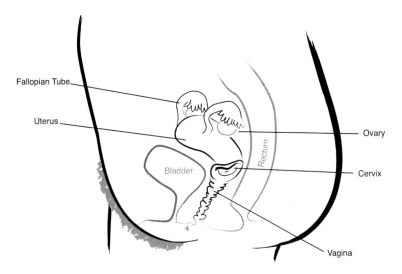

**Figure 1. The internal anatomy of
a woman's reproductive organs**

Kegels are sometimes called "sexercise" because they can improve sensations during love-making. In fact, dads can check the mom's changing muscle strength if she squeezes his penis while having intercourse. Another great benefit of doing Kegels is that they reduce the chance of organ prolapse later in life. Since these muscles are responsible for supporting the uterus, bladder, and rectum, you can see how important keeping them in shape really is!

Another way to condition the vaginal area is through perineal massage. This is a technique that you can do alone or with the assistance of your partner. See Chapter 7 for instructions.

My Aching Back

As the baby descends into your pelvis, your lower back will probably ache. Wearing flat shoes, using good posture, watching your body mechanics (squat, don't bend), sleeping on a hard surface (using pillows for support), and sitting on a birthing ball (which properly aligns your spine) often helps with this discomfort, so does doing pelvic rocking.

Pelvic rocking can be done standing, sitting, side-lying, or on all fours. On all fours, it's often described as trying to arch your back like a scared cat and then relaxing. In the standing, sitting, or side-lying position, it's like thrusting your pelvic bone forward while tucking your buttocks under. Repeat until the pain subsides. Relief is almost instantaneous.

Remembering to change positions frequently toward the end of pregnancy is helpful. Staying in any one position for too long will add to your discomforts. Change your position every hour or so. Try standing, leaning, swaying, kneeling, sitting (in a variety of ways and places), side-lying, semi-reclining, squatting, and on all fours (hands and knees). Using these positions during pregnancy to deal with discomforts will help you to feel confident about using them for pain and progress in your labor.

Positions like squatting and all fours are not commonly used in our society. But both are very beneficial for labor. All fours puts the baby into an anterior position (the best one for birth), and squatting opens up the pelvis (which shortens the birth canal). Practicing these will build your stamina, so you are able to do them longer while in labor. It will also build your comfort in using these positions at your birth, instead of trying them for the first time that day.

You might consider attending special classes or going to other care providers during the pregnancy to help prepare your body and mind. For instance, prenatal exercise or yoga is a wonderful way to stretch and tone the body, while emptying the mind of distractions and learning to relax. Be sure to find an educator who is certified in these areas and discuss your choices with your midwife or doctor. Here's a general rule of thumb: don't begin any new exercise or activity during your pregnancy without checking with your healthcare provider. Most experts agree that walking and swimming are acceptable forms of exercise unless you are told otherwise.

If you use massage or chiropractic to keep your body in shape, be sure the therapist or chiropractor specializes in techniques appropriate for pregnancy. Massage therapists tell us that there are specific acupressure points that may cause miscarriage during pregnancy if stimulated. Your massage therapist would need to be familiar with those areas.

Breasts Have Their Own Brains

We in the baby business swear breasts have their own little brains! We say this because of their many amazing attributes. While you're pregnant, your breasts are actually helping you get ready for the birth.

For instance, the nipples get larger and darker, so the baby can see the bull's-eye better at birth. Also, the Montgomery glands start doing their job during pregnancy. They are the little pimple-like structures on each areola (the part around the nipple) that secrete a special substance that keeps the nipple and areola clean and moist. So you never need to wash or moisturize your nipples and areolas—the secretions do it for you. In fact, using soap on them during pregnancy can actually lead to dryness and cracked or bleeding nipples when the baby starts nursing. Nothing really needs to be done to your breasts to prepare them. Rather, it's what not to do…like rubbing them to toughen them up. That's not really advised these days.

If your nipples get erect when you're wet, that's a good sign. If they seem flat or inverted, the latest recommendation is not to worry about this while you are pregnant. Usually, nursing will help the situation. The key is don't worry. If you need help, a lactation consultant can assist you after your baby is born.

Another impressive thing about your breasts is their ability to help labor along if it hasn't started or slows down. When the nipples are stimulated, a hormone called oxytocin is released, which can cause contractions. This was probably part of the "caveman way" of bringing labor on. Love-making included nipple stimulation and intercourse. Intercourse included ejaculation. In the semen, prostaglandins were present (from the prostate gland) which helped ready the cervix. If the woman had an orgasm, that irritated the uterus, which also contributed to contractions. When women are past their due dates, the caveman way is heartily recommended… even in the 21st century!

If you plan to try other natural means of bringing labor on—massage, herbs, and homeopathy, for instance—make sure you discuss them with your doctor or midwife first.

Speaking of Brains

So far we've talked about getting your body ready for the birth. But getting your mind ready is at least as important.

Human emotions and intelligence are lodged deep within our brains. Preparing for the birth on both levels is important. Emotionally, we need to feel safe, supported, and satisfied. The last couple of chapters have discussed the benefits of both the right human environment and the appropriate support for you. Emotions tell us to seek out those who will offer us the protection and nurturing we desire while birthing and mothering. This is where a blessing way ceremony can really fill an emotional need for an expectant mother.

What Is a Blessing Way?

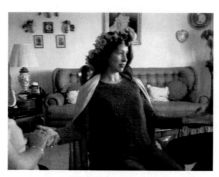

Figure 2. A BlessingWay

Nearly every expectant mom has a baby shower to help her stock up on baby supplies. But how does this prepare the new mother for her birth experience? Becoming a mother is truly a rite of passage. A blessing way is an opportunity to honor the mother, wish her well, and provide spiritual support (Figure 2). It can be religious in nature, but it's often more of the woman-to-woman connection that is celebrated that day. It is fashioned after the Navajo tribal custom of blessing someone's way before an important event—like a wedding, a birth, a war, or a hunt.

What makes a blessing way special is that it's designed with *you* in mind. It's not the usual baby shower with lots of guests, gifts, and games. Only very close female family and friends are invited. No one brings gifts for the baby. Instead, small tokens of affection are brought for the mother-to-be. Tokens can be anything of importance to you or the giver...shells, pins, charms, beads, religious symbols, etc. Cost is unimportant—it's how it makes you feel when you receive it. You can take the tokens (usually in a little bag also from the blessing way) to the birth for additional reassurance and empowerment.

There can be readings, prayers, healing activities, pampering time for the mother, blessings for mom and baby, and special closing words. During the pampering, friends can share positive stories about birth or parenting. A blank journal called a Wisdom Book can be passed around for all to write words of encouragement for the mother. Sometimes, a belly cast (Figure 3) is made during the celebration to capture the beauty of pregnancy and life. Or it's done beforehand, and all who attend the blessing way help to decorate it. The mother could also be blessed by having her pregnant belly decorated by her women friends (Figure 4). All the guests take part in the ceremony. It can last from two hours to nearly all day. At the end, everyone gathers for a potluck feast.

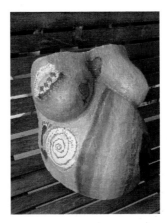

Figure 3. A decorated belly cast

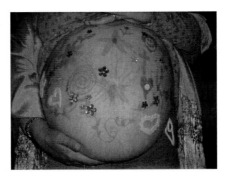

Figure 4. A decorated belly at her blessing way

We have a blessing way for any doula in our group who's pregnant. It starts out being a couple of hours, but often lasts much longer. It's meaningful and special for everyone involved, so we don't want it to end.

A phone chain can be set up to inform all who attended when you are going into labor. That way, you'll be getting all their positive thoughts and vibes when you need them most. A list of who's going to help out at home after the birth can be created to maintain the group's support of you.

A blessing way is another means of returning to the days when women took care of other women around the time of birth. It combines aspects from an ancient culture that celebrated all life had to give with more modern methods of commemorating the miracle of birth.

Does this special celebration appeal to you? Plan one with your close friends.

Ignorance Is Not Always Bliss

Ignorance is not bliss while birthing. Some might think approaching it like the animals do is the way to go. That would be fine if our intellect didn't get in the way of our instincts. Although we should tap into our inner wisdom, strength, and resources as animals do, it seems our human fears stop us from doing just that. We're afraid of the pain, we're afraid of how long it may last, we're afraid of how we'll perform, we're afraid of what the medical experience might be, we're afraid for our health and the baby's, we're afraid of the recovery, we're afraid of parenthood, we're afraid of responsibility, we're afraid of change. We're just plain afraid, and that leads to vulnerability.

Instead of going with the flow of birth, we humans tend to doubt our ability and rely on others to get us through. We sometimes actually add to our own feelings of helplessness that normally occur during a birth. Why go there, as they say? Arming yourself with good information, good support, and good attitudes will help you find the innate ability in you.

Think Creatively: Use Your Right Brain

Long before they hit the slopes, Olympic skiers picture themselves skiing down the course—making course corrections, determining how they will move their body, visualizing what the obstacles will be and how to best get around the obstacles, and planning how they will make a winning run. This thinking work actually helps their bodies physically prepare. You can use this technique when you visualize your birth before labor begins.

Have someone read this visualization activity to you. Try not to do anything physical during your visualization. Don't intensify your breathing or practice pushing. Just picture your birth smoothly happening. Studies have shown that these kinds of visualizations work as practice for your body.

Birth Visualization Activity:

1. Sit in a comfortable position in a quiet room.

2. Close your eyes and visualize that your baby is in the head-down (vertex) position, ready to be born.

3. You feel a contraction come, and you are able to relax into the contraction, working with it, allowing it to open up your cervix slowly and surely.

4. Your baby slowly moves lower in your pelvis, getting closer and closer to being born.

5. Your contractions come, one at a time. You are able to cope with each one as it comes. You are able to relax and breathe during the contraction. You rest between contractions.

6. Every once in a while, you change positions to help gravity guide your baby lower, closer to birth.

7. Finally, your baby is low enough for you to feel the urge to push. You push naturally, with your body's urges. Each push brings your baby lower, closer to being born and placed in your arms.

8. Your pushes gently open you, stretching your skin slowly. Then your baby's head is born. Next, your baby's shoulders and body are born. Your baby is here!

Now that you have pictured your baby's birth, think about the circumstances that made the birth a comfortable environment for you. Was the room dark or bright? Who was around you, giving you support? Did your supporters speak encouragements to you or was there silence? Was there soft music playing? Were there any pleasing scents in the air? What sort of room did you give birth in? How long did you think your birth would take? Was there anything that was important to you that you found comforting? Think about the answers and make a mental note of them. You can use this visualization many times if you wish.

Birth is also emotional. While giving birth, you will open yourself up both physically and emotionally. You will need emotional support while you do your wonderful birth work. Here is a quiz to get you started thinking about what support you prefer.

What Supports You Emotionally – Quiz

Circle all that apply.

1. I like to have quiet and privacy when I'm trying to relax.

2. I enjoy having constant reminders and encouragement to help me cope.

3. I feel more calm when I listen to calming music.

4. I like to pray or chant when I am dealing with stress.

5. It is easy for me to picture a safe and relaxing place – like a beach.

6. Affirmations help me stay positive.

7. I know I can achieve difficult things, because I have overcome important obstacles in the past.

8. I feel comfortable with dim lighting and a calm environment.

9. I feel more energized and at home when the lights are bright and the music is upbeat.

10. The calm tone of someone's voice helps me focus on staying relaxed.

11. I like to be kept informed of everything because that helps me stay calm and in control.

12. Counting helps me get through small events.

13. I enjoy listening to my baby's heartbeat on the monitor.

14. Listening to my baby's heartbeat for a long time would make me anxious.

Partner's assistance:

Think of three times in your past when you know she was very strong and overcame big difficulties. Keep these to yourself, so that you can remind her of how strong she was at the crucial moment during her labor.

Chapter 12 will help you create a written birth vision of your own to share with your birth team. Your birth vision will include the preferences you have identified here. Ideally, your birth vision will include things that support you both physically and emotionally.

In the Hospital Things Go Beep!

If you are going to give birth in a hospital, keep in mind that things will go beep! There are monitors, IV infusers—even machines in other rooms that you might hear. It can be distracting. Be prepared for sounds and interruptions. Have your own soothing, calming music with you. It will help you stay in your birthing groove and keep your focus. It will also make the room more relaxing for nurses who come in to check on you. When your nurse is more relaxed, she will be another calming member of your birth team. If your baby's heart rate is being monitored, you will hear it. Some women are reassured to hear it, and some prefer to have the sound turned down.

Going Back to School

You've already learned about good support and attitudes in the preceding chapters. Good information is the last piece of the puzzle. Education is the only way to learn what you need to know, so it's back to school! Education should occur before, during, and after the birth. There are so many ways to learn these days (Table 3).

Table 3. Ways to Learn

SELF	PEER	FORMAL	CASUAL
reading	family	classes	acquaintances
internet	old friends	HCP appointments	new friends
TV	support groups	conferences	chat sites

And there is a cornucopia of classes available:

- Early Pregnancy
- Childbirth Preparation
- Breastfeeding
- Baby Care
- Infant & Child First Aid
- Infant & Child CPR
- Infant Massage
- Sibling Class

Where's the Ice Chip Machine?

Taking a tour of the birthing facility (whether it be a birth center or a hospital) can be helpful and reassuring. That way, you know where to go, what to bring, and what to expect. You can also learn something about the facility's protocols and procedures. You'll feel much more comfortable, and there will be fewer surprises.

Making sure a visiting sibling feels okay with mommy and baby's new environment is another consideration. A class to orient the sibling to the facility is a great idea. Aside from receiving the buttons, balloons, coloring book, and snack, the sibling learns where you will be while away from home and what babies are about. Knowing cafeteria and gift-shop details is also a good idea when dealing with siblings. Having a family member take the older sibling to the gift ship to buy baby a present is fun. And running down to the cafeteria to get an ice cream cone to celebrate the new baby's birth can turn a cranky kid into a happy child. It's always nice to get the older sibling a gift from the baby as well. We just expect the older child to adapt and accept this new sister or brother willingly and lovingly. A little present from the baby will help with this transition.

The Other Kids

For many of us, pets are really the first kids before a human baby arrives. Including them in the preparation for the baby's homecoming is probably a good idea. Keeping the nursery room door closed, never letting them sniff baby items, separating them from you, and changing usual habits is confusing to pets. They are curious and interested and want to be with you. They sense something is about to happen...like an earthquake coming to change their lives!

Be sure your pets are healthy and well behaved before bringing baby home. *Never leave any pet alone with your baby.* Keeping doors closed is easy with baby monitors. Gates can also keep unwanted pets out of a room, as well as a screen door. If you're concerned about your cat getting into the baby's crib or bassinet, just line it with aluminum foil or fill it with blown-up balloons. A cat who jumps onto either of those will get scared and won't return. And remember to bring a baby item home for the pet to smell before bringing the baby home. When you come home, mom should greet the pet with open arms, and dad should carry the baby in. Let the pet smell and interact with the baby, so the connection can be made and the pet's curiosity satisfied.

Tying up Loose Ends

The way to feel prepared for the birth is to consider all that defines you, affects you, and surrounds you. That's why we included sections in this chapter about everything from your pelvic floor to pets. Feeling informed through education is important, but feeling like all is ready for the baby is vital, as well. Being ready, prepared, organized, focused, centered, and primed for the big event and all it entails afterwards will result in a better outcome for your family. Adjustments are easier to make when you know what to expect and what helps.

To help you feel more informed and prepared, we've included labor bag suggestions, a pregnancy checklist, and a physical support questionnaire at the end of this chapter. They will expand your knowledge, guide your actions, and help you make your decisions. Enjoy!

LABOR BAG

Consider packing:

- Camera(s)/film/battery
- Tape/CD/MP3 player, batteries, and music
- Aromatherapy (lavender, mint, and citrus are generally non-offensive)
- Plastic spoons and straws
- Snacks/drinks (for both)
- Lip balm/lip gloss (unflavored)
- Sour lollipops/candy sticks (sugar = energy)
- Mouthwash or breath freshener
- Fan (hand or battery operated/batteries)
- Instant cold pack/ice wrap
- Brush/hair ties
- Hot water bottle/instant hot pack
- Rice sock (microwave on high for 3 minutes.)
- Small spritzer bottle (fill with plain/scented water to refresh body/room)
- Socks (red so bodily fluids aren't so noticeable)
- Massage cream/lotion/corn starch
- Wooden/textured/vibrating massagers
- Tennis ball (for massage)
- 2 Stress balls (for hand massage)
- 2 Small pocket combs (for acupressure points on palms)
- Soft stuffed animal (for comforting tactile stimulation)
- Sea Bands (for nausea)
- Mirror (to view baby's head)

- Focal point(s)
- Kneeling pads
- Birth Vision (make available to staff)
- Paper/pen
- Parking/meal $
- Phone list/phone card
- Notes – Labor & Breastfeeding
- Religious/cultural/personal items

Also Bring:
- Birthing Ball
- Bed/body pillows (NOT in white cases)
- Mom's clothes for labor/personal belongings
- Change of clothes/swimsuit for partner

Additional supplies for doulas:
- Rebozo (Mexican shawl)
- White noise machine
- Aromatherapy diffuser
- Business cards/brochures/client paperwork

PREGNANCY CHECKLIST

Use this as a checklist to keep track of considerations regarding the birth.

√	Put a checkmark if you've handled the specific consideration and jot down details beside it.
	Choose your birth place [home, birth center, hospital]
	Choose your healthcare providers [midwife or doctor]
	Choose your birth team [partner, mother, family member, or close friend]
	Hire a birth doula; consider need for postpartum doula
	Attend classes [childbirth, breastfeeding, infant CPR, infant care, infant massage]
	Work through birth concerns [visualizations, journaling, art]
	Write your birth vision [philosophy, preferences, priorities]
	Prepare for changes to your home and work [supplies, arrangements, support]
	Contact local Le Leche League group(free breastfeeding support group), attend meeting: see breastfeeding babies and meet other women
	Treat yourself [yoga, exercise, nutrition/cooking, massage/relaxation, manicure/pedicure]
	Fun activity with friends and family [lunch dates, movies, picnic]
	Special moments with partner [date or intimate evening]

What Supports You Physically – Quiz

Here are some ideas and suggestions for what you may find comforting during labor. Circle your favorite answer to each question.

1. When you are feeling sick or injured, do you feel more comfortable –

    a.   Quietly alone in a dim room to curl up by yourself.

    b.   In a dim room with quiet music by yourself.

    c.   In a bright room with a loved one bringing you something to eat or massaging you. Daylight makes you feel more comfortable.

    d.   With lots of activity around jollying you out of feeling bad.

2. While trying to relax you like to –

    a.   Listen to quiet music on headphones.

    b.   Listen to guided meditations or self-hypnosis.

    c.   Enjoy calming aromatherapy, like lavender or other scents.

    d.   Be massaged or touched gently.

    e.   Take a warm bath or shower.

3. When you picture yourself in labor, what rhythms would be soothing to you –

    a.   Rocking in a rocking chair or on a birth ball.

    b.   Standing and swaying.

    c.   Counting until the contraction is over.

    d.   Dancing to tribal music.

4. What areas do you like to be touched or massaged –

    a.   Hands or feet

    b.   Neck and shoulders

    c.   Head

    d.   Anywhere I want to relieve stress and pain.

5. What areas do you find ticklish or prefer not to be touched –

   a. Massage doesn't usually relax me, I'm very ticklish

   b. Feet

   c. Back

   d. Side or lower back

6. When you are at home, what comforts you that you might be able to bring to your birth place? –

   a. Big shirt or robe.

   b. Pillowcase that smells like home.

   c. Special light food or drink (which your doctor approves).

   d. Special soft stuffed animal (or photo of beloved pet).

   e. Your favorite soothing (wordless) music.

If you have three or more a or b answers, you are more inwardly focused and prefer quiet to bustle when you are trying to cope with labor. Your birth vision should focus on how you would like the atmosphere to reflect your need for quiet.

If you have three or more c answers, you like more active help, and you like to be more active yourself. You enjoy engaging all of your senses to help you cope with labor, this includes, scent, counting, and some massage.

If you have three or more d or e answers, you are more outwardly focused and have an easier time accepting help. Your focus is more on getting support where you need it (in the form of a massage or a warm bath) than the need for quiet concentration.

If you had trouble narrowing your choices, that is ok! During different parts of labor, you may be comforted by different techniques and atmospheres. You might try starting with a quiet atmosphere during early labor to help you adjust to your new environment and have more light or a warm bath later when you are in active labor. Use all of these as suggestions for what you might like to support you during labor.

Chapter 5

When Labor Begins

Lena was heavily pregnant. It was just a few days until her due date. Some days she felt like just waddling around the house was all the exercise she needed. Then one morning, she awoke with a renewed purpose. How could she bring a baby into this house? She realized that her door knobs and door hinges were filthy, the closet in the nursery wasn't organized, and the vents hadn't been cleaned in forever. She had to fix it all right now! Once the baby was born, she wouldn't have time to do it.

Luckily, she felt energized for the task. She started with the dirtiest door hinges and knobs. To really clean them she had to unscrew them and put them in the dishwasher. Four of her doors were the worst offenders. While the dishwasher churned, she vacuumed the vents, sometimes standing on a chair to reach them. Then she pulled everything out of the nursery closet and wiped it down, and then vacuumed. She assembled a hanging closet organizer.

When her husband Jeff got home, Lena was struggling to hold a door in place while she rehung it. Jeff gasped, "What the heck are you doing?" He sat her down to rest and rehung the doors himself. The next day, their baby girl was born.

Changes Leading up to the Big Day

Pregnancy lasts about 280 days - give or take 2 weeks in either direction. Leading up to your due date, you'll notice changes. The baby will lighten or "drop," sometimes up to a month before the baby comes. You'll have different discomforts now, and that tells you the baby is moving down. Instead of shortness of breath and indigestion, you'll have lower backache and make more trips to the bathroom. This means frequent toilet breaks during the night. We say this is Mother Nature's way of preparing you for being up every few hours after the baby arrives.

Pelvic rocking, good posture, sitting on the birth ball, wearing flat shoes, a firm sleeping surface, appropriate body mechanics, and hydrotherapy all help the backache. When the birth is near, many women feel a "fullness" deep within their hips, which is a good sign that the baby has settled in the pelvis. Squatting can help relieve that sensation if it's bothering you. Sitting on the ball and making circles, rocking, swaying, or bouncing is another great way to feel more comfortable when your pelvis aches. You can also adjust the baby by using the apron lift (see Chapter 6) for comfort. Remember, this loosening of the pelvis is what allows the baby to fit through, so feel good about your body doing its job. Getting into the hands-and-knees position can encourage the baby into an anterior position before birth, which can also reduce pelvic discomfort. Why not put her into the best position for you both leading into the birth?

A healthy-sized baby is more crowded toward the end of your pregnancy, so the baby may not move as often. Your midwife or doctor will advise you as to how to keep track of movement. Ten movements in twelve hours is often the standard. If you're concerned, call your care provider.

Contractions will change from stretching the uterus to shrinking the uterus. The *stretching* contractions, called Braxton-Hicks, allow for the individual muscle fibers of the uterus to stretch to accommodate the growing baby. As labor begins, the uterine muscles shorten, which causes the uterus to shrink—forcing the baby out. Braxton-Hicks can get regular enough that some women go to the place of birth too early. Unless cervical changes accompany the contractions, it is not true labor.

When you feel contractions, try changing your activity or taking a shower. If the contractions continue, it could be labor. If they stop, it wasn't.

Most care providers tell women to call them when contractions are 3-5 minutes apart, lasting 60 seconds, for at least an hour. This can mean you'll be in active labor upon arrival at the birth place. You may not be able to walk and talk through those contractions, which is a good sign that you're working hard.

Remember:

- *How far apart your contractions are* is measured from the *beginning* of one to the *beginning* of the next.

- *How long each contraction lasts* is measured from the beginning of the contraction to the end.

When you talk to your healthcare providers, they'll want both those measurements.

CAUTION: If you are *less than 37 weeks* pregnant and contractions occur every 15 minutes or so for 2 hours, call your care provider. It could be preterm labor. Lying flat on your left side and drinking lots of water is often suggested to slow the contractions. This is because lying on your left side is an anti-gravity position and, when you drink a lot of water, it goes into the bloodstream and dilutes the hormone oxytocin, which causes contractions. You can also dilute the oxytocin by taking a warm bath. The water pressure forces fluids from your tissues into the bloodstream, reducing the oxytocin.

Another sign that labor may be beginning is diarrhea. We call it Mother Nature's enema. It's your body's method of clearing the way for the baby. You may also not feel very hungry the day you go into labor, which should be a really big tip that something is different.

Your Body Is Getting Ready

Keep in mind, your due date is a guideline, not a promise. Closer to your due date, you'll see an increase in your vaginal discharge. It's your body's way of cleansing and lubricating the birth canal for the baby. Many women start wearing a panty liner the last month to stay cleaner and dryer. Since the baby is putting pressure on your bladder after dropping, urinary leakage is not unusual...especially if you cough, sneeze, or laugh! The panty liner helps with that, as well.

Some moms see their mucus plug before going into labor. The cervix has opened enough to allow the plug (which provided protection during pregnancy) to be released. The dilation causes cervical capillaries to break, which streaks the mucus with pink, red, or brown. Although it isn't a direct sign of labor, we say, "Be sure your bags are packed!" If you are past your due date, you'll be looking for that particular sign. We often see labor within a couple of days of losing the plug, but it could be weeks. A lot of women don't see their plug because it comes out in bits and pieces or gets flushed late at night when lights aren't on.

Even Your Breasts Are Revving up

You may have a yellowish discharge from your nipples called colostrum. This is the liquid gold the baby will get every time she nurses until your milk comes in about the third to fifth day after birth. Even though it is a limited amount, colostrum is thick and rich in fat and calories, so it satisfies the baby's nutritional needs perfectly. Just continue to keep your breasts clean with water. Don't use soap— it can cause dryness. It's nice to know your baby will get this liquid gold right away.

She's Hosing Down the Aluminum Siding!

Ever heard of the nesting instinct? You may find yourself feeling driven to get your home ready for the baby's arrival. It can be something as simple as making casseroles to freeze for postpartum dinners, or it can be hosing down the aluminum siding.

But do try to avoid doing any activity that will tire you, since you may be going into labor soon. Fight the urge to do something big, and direct your energy to readying yourself for the birth. Think about the first nest the baby will see and build that place wherever you decide to give birth. Gather the personal stuff that will make your birth area your own, and start mentally preparing for the exciting event.

This Is It—Or Is It?

If your water breaks or your contractions meet the criteria mentioned above, call the doctor or midwife. Calling when you lose your plug is not usually suggested, but mentioning it at an appointment is quite appropriate. Whatever cervical changes occur before labor actually begins, that's less you have to do during labor. So, be sure to ask about cervical direction (posterior or anterior), effacement (measured in per cent), dilation (measured in centimeters), baby's station (plus or minus), and baby's position (anterior or posterior) whenever you're examined. Get all the facts!

Many changes occur to the cervix as it readies for the birth. During pregnancy, it is facing towards your back (posterior) for additional protection for the baby. As you approach your due date, it moves towards your front (anterior), so the baby can more easily move through the pelvis and down the vaginal birth canal.

The cervix also ripens which means it goes from being hard to soft, like a peach as it ripens. Feel your forehead, then the tip of your nose, and then your earlobe. This feels like the process of cervical softening.

Once it ripens, the cervix can then efface or thin. The cervix is normally about 2 inches in length. As it shortens while thinning, a percentage of effacement is assigned according to how much is gone. So, if the cervix is 1 inch long, that would be 50% effacement. If it is a ½ inch long, the effacement is 75%.

Once effacement begins, dilation generally follows. Dilation is how much the cervix actually opens (from 0 to 10 centimeters or about 4 inches). This seems to be the most important reading to staff during exams, but so much more can be determined during those 30 seconds or so.

Be sure to ask what other changes have occurred if there has been no change in your dilation. It seems to take a long time to get to 5 centimeters because your cervix is completing effacement, as well. Once your cervix is 5 centimeters dilated and fully effaced, the rest of your dilation usually happens quickly.

Another issue is the baby's station. That is where the baby's head is in relation to the narrowest diameter of your pelvis. If the baby is 1 centimeter above that point, the station is -1 (minus one). Even with that point, 0 station. One centimeter beyond that point would be +1 (plus one), and so forth. The baby crowns at +4 or +5 station, which means it no longer retreats back into your body between pushes and birth is near. If the baby does not make it into the + numbers, a cesarean birth is indicated.

The last measurement that can be determined during an exam is the baby's position. Is the hard back of the head (called the occiput) in front or is it pressing on your spine in back? We want the baby to be facing your spine, so its soft fleshy face doesn't hurt your back as it descends. Plus, the baby senses the arch of the pubic bone behind its neck to lift, extend, and birth its head. So, it's important for the baby's back to be toward the front of your body. If it is, we call that anterior. If the baby is posterior, it results in painful back labor, since the boney head is pushing against the bones of your spine.

This is the most common complication in first time births, but it can be corrected pretty easily during labor using position changes, certain tools, and specific techniques. Backache is the main indicator that your baby is posterior in the earlier parts of labor. At the end of labor, many women have some discomfort as the baby pushes their tail bone out of the way during Second Stage.

You may be able to put the baby in the anterior position before your birth to avoid back labor. This can be done by leaning forward while sitting or while standing. You can also do this by leaning over the ball while on hands and knees, so gravity pulls the back of the baby's hard head towards the floor (which also means to the front of your body). Doing these three things (for several minutes at a time) about 2 weeks before your due date can really be helpful. Also, try not to become a hammock for your baby by slumping back into the sofa, for instance. And remember, sitting on the birth ball during pregnancy really helps to align your spine, thus reducing many discomforts associated with the end of gestation.

If you followed the 5-1-1 rule about going to the birth facility, you might hear measurements like these: cervix is midway, 80% effacement, 3 centimeters dilation, minus one station with baby in an anterior position. If you wait until your contractions are three minutes apart, you will probably be more like anterior cervix, 100% effaced, 4-5 centimeters dilated, and baby at a zero station and in the anterior position. We want both the cervix and baby to be anterior (not posterior). It pays to stay home longer if possible so labor is well established when you arrive.

If your water breaks when labor begins, take note of these things: when it happened, whether it was a gush or a trickle, what the color was, and whether you're contracting. Call your care provider and follow their directions.

The great majority of women experience their water breaking during active or transitional labor, well after contractions have begun. Time is an issue, since the chance of infection increases after the sac ruptures. As doulas, we've seen doctors wanting babies *born* within 24 hours after the water breaks. With midwives, we see them wanting *contractions* within 24 hours. That's a big difference, so be sure to discuss this with your care provider.

More about Those Birth Fluids

Even if your water breaks with a gush, you won't have a dry labor. The sac continues to make fluid until the placenta comes out.

A gush is pretty obvious, since it's about a quart of fluid. If it's a trickle, it's hard to know. We often suggest wearing a pad and seeing if it keeps getting wet. If you smell it and it smells like ammonia, it's urine. If it smells sweet, it's amniotic fluid. You can also do a Kegel. That will stop urine, but not amniotic fluid. Your midwife or doctor can do easy tests to determine for sure whether your water has broken.

The color is important to note. It should be clear or slightly straw colored. If it is green, brown, or black, tell your care provider and expect to go right to the hospital. It means the baby has had a short period of oxygen deprivation and has released its first bowel movement into the fluid. The lack of oxygen causes the muscles in the rectum to relax and release the meconium. You will be consistently monitored during the birth to watch for a repeat of this situation.

After your water breaks, whenever that is, you may notice little squirts during contractions. Once the bag of water is gone, so is the protective aspect of the sac.

Infection is now more likely, so internal exams are limited and only sterile gloves are used. Your movements may be limited, which could affect your ability to change positions freely. Antibiotics may be ordered if infection is a concern.

If your water breaks and the baby's station is high, your care provider will be concerned about cord prolapse. If the water gushes, and the baby's head is high in the pelvis, the cord could get swept down in front of the baby's head and get compressed. Your baby is getting all her oxygen from her cord, so cord prolapse is a very serious complication, although it is very, very rare (it happens in fewer than 1% of births).

If your care provider suggests breaking your water to speed up labor, you may want to pause a moment and consider the consequences. Once it is broken, there is no going back. You *must* give birth. A countdown has now begun: your labor will only be allowed to continue for so long. After the sac is gone, the baby's hard head feels quite different from a bulging bag of water against the cervix—so it generally hurts more during the contraction. Then you might feel the need for pain medication, when in fact you might not have needed it at all if the water hadn't been broken. In addition, an intact sac cushions your baby's head. Without the sac, your baby's head will feel uneven pressure.

There are times when breaking the water is a good idea. For example, if you are in transition, and your bag is bulging, breaking your water will allow the baby to finish dilating the cervix. This is the time when the sac commonly breaks anyway. Or it may be necessary to break the water to check the color of the fluid because the staff suspects stress. Always ask what the medical indication is, and accept it if you are satisfied with the answer. If you make an informed decision, you will feel good about your choices during and after the birth.

Will You Have a "Textbook Average" Birth?

Although every labor is different, there are some generalizations that can be used as a guide. Table 4 shows how labor often progresses from First Stage (dilation of the cervix) to Second Stage (pushing the baby out) to Third Stage (delivery of the placenta). We call this a "textbook average" guide for birth.

Table 4. Labor & Birth

Stage 1 – Labor			
Phases:	**Early**	**Active**	**Transition**
Time:	7 hours	5 hours	1 hour
Dilation:	0-4 centimeters	4-8 centimeters	8-10 centimeters
Frequency	20-25 minutes	5 to 3 minutes	2 minutes
Duration:	30-45 seconds	45-60 seconds	90 seconds
Stage 2 –Birth			
Time:	30 minutes to 3 hours		
Dilation:	10 centimeters		
Frequency:	3 minutes		
Duration:	60 seconds		
Stage 3 – Placenta			
Expelled:	15-30 minutes after baby is born		

Questions About Progress:

1. What direction is my cervix facing? (goes from posterior to anterior)

2. How much cervical effacement? (goes from 0 to 100 %)

3. How much cervical dilation? (goes from 0 to 10 cms.)

4. What is the baby's station? (goes from minus to plus numbers)

5. What is the baby's position? (anterior is preferable to posterior)

You can ask these questions individually or you can simply ask: "What other changes have occurred?" Keep in mind that dilation isn't everything.

Go Later Rather than Sooner

During early labor, pass the time doing usual activities like going to work, eating, and shopping with a friend or taking in a movie. If you stay home, watch a good DVD, listen to your favorite CD, bake your favorite kind of cookies, take a relaxing bath, or do a small job. Remember to rest or sleep if you can. Make sure you drink plenty of fluids and eat lightly and regularly. Ask your partner for a nice back or foot massage. See how your doctor or midwife feels about having you come in later rather than sooner.

Every woman is different, and every labor is different. You and your care provider will have to decide when is the right time for *you* to come to the birth place. These are some of the things you'll have to take into account:

- last visit's statistics (direction of cervix, effacement, dilation, station)
- which baby this is (first usually takes longer)
- current conditions (status of amniotic fluid, contraction characteristics, and your pain level)
- your own emotional state (some mothers need support sooner than others)
- distance to the birthplace and weather or traffic conditions

Since it takes a while to get to 5 centimeters, why not stay home and remain in control for as long as you can? This is why we often recommend that you not rush to the hospital. Don't set yourself up to *turn into a patient* by arriving too early. Remember that you are *not sick* when you're in labor. Quite the contrary—your body is doing what it was intended to do.

Chapter 6
Active Labor

When the doula arrived, Adele and her husband, Jim, were in a triage room. Her contractions were already strong. Adele was crying and saying, "I can't do this! I need an epidural!" The pain made her feel out of control and lost.

Her doula told her she could have an epidural if she needed one, but not in triage. "Let's get you out of bed and onto the birth ball first."

While Adele sat on the ball and bounced, Jim and her doula each took hold of one of her hands to massage.

Adele was no longer crying, but she still felt like she wasn't coping well. She said: "I can't do this!" several times between her contractions.

Her doula noticed that during a contraction, Adele would close her eyes tight, feeling overwhelmed. What she needed was focus—focus on the task at hand, not on her pain and her fear.

The doula asked Jim if they had brought a focal point for Adele. He worriedly admitted they didn't have one. So her doula took a photo of a baby out of her bag and told Adele to look at the baby during her contractions. For several contractions, Adele bounced on the ball, while Jim and her doula massaged her hands, and she focused on the picture of the baby. Things were still feeling intense, but better than before.

During the next contraction, her doula had Adele say together with her: "*Hhhhh* I can do it! *Hhhhh* I can do it!" over and over. The "*hhhhh*" helped Adele keep her jaw open and relaxed, which helped her open and relax her perineum. The "I can do it!" started as just something to say together, but as Adele kept getting through each contraction one by one, she became calmer and more assured. She slowly started to realize that she *was* doing it! Her doula had helped her layer one coping strategy on another during each contraction, and those strategies were working together to help her feel calm and focus on the birth.

Soon, the nurse came back and took Adele into her labor room. Her doctor checked her cervix and found she was almost fully dilated and nearly ready to push. Adele kept coping with her husband's and doula's help. She never asked for an epidural again—even though she could have had one if she had wanted one. After her beautiful boy was born, she realized she *had* done it! No one could ever take that accomplishment away from her.

It Takes a Long Time to Get to 5 Centimeters

Remember those words. About two thirds of the birth process is getting into good, active labor. By reminding yourself that it will take a while to get halfway in dilation, it will help you stay focused on normal progress. You won't feel worried about having the stamina to make it through another 10 or 12 hours. Ask your partner to tell you that frequently in labor. Always keeping the right perspective is a big part of staying positive during the birth.

Active labor is the perfect term for when labor intensifies. Your body gets more active, your birth team gets more active. Active labor is usually tolerable for most moms with contractions probably being 3-5 minutes apart and 60+ seconds long. Your cervix finishes effacement and works towards complete dilation from 4 to 10 centimeters. Your baby continues to twist and turn its way down and out.

The Amazing Cervix

After most women get to 5 centimeters, things seem to move quickly. The cervix thins and opens more readily. Moms tend to get serious about the contractions. They need to concentrate on coping skills more than before and can begin to doubt their ability to handle it. If you can welcome the pain, absorb it, and work with it, labor will flow better. If you are scared of the pain, fight it, and resist the contraction, labor will suffer – not to mention you! Let the cervix open – open – open. Doulas often use imagery of something opening or blossoming, while whispering "open" during labor. It's the power of suggestion at work.

The cervix is one of the body's many sphincters. A sphincter is a ring-shaped muscle that surrounds a natural opening in the body and can open or close by expanding or contracting. According to midwife Ina May Gaskin's Sphincter Law, she firmly believes that the cervical sphincter is shy, doesn't obey commands, and responds well to praise, smiling, and laughter. She also recognizes the important connection between the open mouth and the open cervix, and the relaxed jaw and the relaxed sphincter.

How Do You Know if It's Active Labor?

Sometimes it's hard to tell if you are in active labor yet. Many books suggest that active labor is four or more centimeters dilated. That's only a starting point, not the whole story. In active labor, you will feel the need to move around to cope with contractions. Sitting or lying still won't be comfortable. Your cervix will be making changes. It may move anterior, efface further, or dilate. The baby's station may move lower, as well. You should see some changes in three to five hours. If you don't see changes, you are still in the latent phase of labor.

To Feel or Not to Feel - That Is the Question

Active labor is when the majority of women accepting drugs have them. Narcotics and regional anesthesia are available. Narcotics commonly offered include Nubain and Stadol. They are intended to increase your tolerance to the pain or "take the edge off." You can still feel the contraction, but are able to cope better and rest better, if you couldn't before. Consider having half a dose to see if it works for you. You can always ask for the other half, if you feel you need more. However, once a whole dose is in, you can't take it out. We never know how drugs will individually affect women in labor, so have the least amount first. Here's a list of more considerations before accepting drugs of any kind:

Hints on Knowing if and When Drugs Are Needed:

- If you are not sure you need drugs, then you probably don't.

- Try not to predict the need for drugs by anticipating increasing pain.

- Make an effort not to let the availability of drugs or their frequent offering influence you.

- Support person - don't confuse her coping with suffering from the pain. The ultimate decision is hers.

- Consider making a pact to wait an agreed upon length of time (20-30 minutes) to try labor coping skills again.

- As a quick review of labor coping skills, the birth team can check PURRRR:

  - P-Position: is she changing position every half hour?

  - U-Urination: is she voiding every hour?

  - R-Relaxation: Is she as relaxed as possible?

  - R-Respiration: Is she breathing evenly (inhalation = exhalation)?

  - R-Rest: Is she taking advantage of the built in breaks?

  - R-Reassurance: Is she feeling encouraged and supported?

- Ask to be checked to determine dilation before accepting drugs, so you can make an informed decision.

- Ask for a review of possible side-effects on mother, baby, and labor, and ask about other birthing coping strategies.

Timing is everything when it comes to narcotics. That's why you always want to have a cervical exam before accepting drugs. It may not be an appropriate time for you, the labor, or the baby. Having Stadol or Nubain too close to the actual birth can cause respiratory distress for the baby. This can affect the baby's apgar scoring (quick medical assessment at 1 and 5 minutes after birth) and your immediate interaction with him, which effects bonding and breastfeeding. No drug used in obstetrics today has been shown to be 100% safe, so feel sure that you need it before accepting it.

The Epidural Epidemic

We are seeing the unprecedented use of epidurals in the great majority of American births these days. It truly is of epidemic proportions when hospitals report epidural rates at 80 to 90% (or even higher). Why are so many women using them? Has their ability to deal with labor suddenly diminished in the last several decades? For hundreds of thousands of years, women gave birth with no drugs, but relied on their own natural pain relief called endorphins.

Many of us in the baby business feel it's due to several reasons:

- Society is into high tech (must be the best).

- Society is into quick fixes (very little patience).

- Society equates pain with pathology (something being wrong).

- Society defines birth as a way to expand the family (not as an essential rite of passage).

- Society lacks a real confidence in the body (and its innate ability to do its job).

- Doctors and staff are recommending them. (Why feel pain if you don't have to?)

- Friends and family also recommend them. (It will validate their decision to have an epidural if you do as well. Or it will make the birth easier for them … if it works.)

- Educators sometimes don't realistically prepare mothers to have a drug-free childbirth (classes are more of a hospital orientation).

- Insurance companies are readily paying for them. (Would you pay the $1500 if the insurance company wouldn't?)

- Women often lack the confidence to try it naturally (no previous hospitalizations, no real pain history, no real support from loved ones or caretakers, no real knowledge on how to cope or even why she should).

That brings up the epidural questions. So, what is it, why is it used, when should it be done, how is it done, who does it, and where is it done?

How to Know When to Say Yes

Asking yourself the questions mentioned above is the first step in deciding what you'll have and when you'll have it. Understanding what an epidural is and what it entails is part of the decision process. An epidural is a form of a regional anesthetic. It can be used for either a vaginal or cesarean birth. It is administered through a hollow needle and catheter arrangement in the lumbar section of the spine into the epidural space. The dural sac is what holds the spinal fluid. An epidural means the medication is put into the area outside (epi) of the dural sac. The medications used are a mixture of drugs, the essential one being a type of "caine" medication. This is like novacaine used in the dentist's office. You feel the sensations of him working in your mouth, but not the sensations of the pain when drilling, for example. A "caine" medication blocks the pain sensation from traveling along the nerve pathways to the brain. No message to the brain, no feeling of pain for the person.

If the epidural is done well and correctly, the recipient should be able to move a bit, but not feel contraction pain. Epidurals are technically difficult to administer, and sometimes they just don't work as expected. Women complain of the epidural being lop-sided, still feeling the contraction, but in a different place, or getting no relief at all. These are unfortunate, especially when you are counting on it to work so you can get some rest, but it doesn't. Accepting an epidural also means accepting:

- Staying in bed (reduced movement)
- Urinating on a bedpan (or being catheterized)
- Constant IV (keep your blood pressure up)
- Constant blood pressure cuff (epidurals are known for reducing your blood pressure)
- Constant monitoring (external or internal)
- Possibly:
    - A pulse oxymeter (to check mom's oxygenation)
    - Pitocin (to augment contractions)
    - Additional medication (to increase your blood pressure)
    - Longer pushing (often can't feel to push)
    - Oxygen mask (to ensure a good flow of oxygen to baby)
    - Episiotomy (to speed up pushing)
    - Instrument delivery (to help baby out)
    - Cesarean birth (often due to "failure to progress")

Avoid an Epidural Fever

Getting an epidural often makes a woman hot, even feverish. If you develop a fever during labor, your baby will be carefully evaluated for fever, as well. A hot mommy often produces a baby who is feverish at birth. Unfortunately, fevers in newborns have to be taken seriously because if your baby had an infection, he could become seriously ill. Doctors don't have the luxury to wait several days for an infection to develop, they must assume that a feverish baby may have an infection and treat with antibiotics.

To avoid this, do not bundle up with blankets after receiving an epidural. Instead, make the room cooler and have only a sheet covering you. If you start to feel at all hot, get cold compresses on your forehead and wrists. Keep your temperature down, and you can usually avoid an epidural fever.

Really Picking up Steam Now

The phase of labor right before pushing called transition is usually the hardest to handle. Long, strong, and close contractions dilate your cervix from 8 to 10 centimeters. Moms can experience sweating, trembling, vomiting, and increased bloody show in response to intense transitional changes. Fatigue and doubt, which can produce anxiety, also present a challenge. It's normal for women to be swept away emotionally when feeling overwhelmed physically. But transition is also the shortest phase, and because you're busy coping with contractions, it tends to go quickly. It is, however, when most women feel it's time for drugs, but it is often too late. The drugs either won't have time to take effect or will have a negative effect on the baby. It's natural to worry about being able to maintain the necessary stamina and power to do this awesome job! That's why you surround yourself with constructive and positive people.

Sometimes the mom will get an urge to bear down before complete dilation, say at 9 or 9+ centimeters. It is not how dilated you are that gives you the urge to push, it is how low your baby's head is within your pelvis. Follow your midwife's or doctor's advice on how to proceed. We find that relieving the urge with baby pushes or grunts will often encourage the rest of the cervix to dilate, but not tear or swell. Hospital staff often has you blow the urge away until complete. It will prevent you from pushing. This can confuse some women about coordinating their efforts when they are allowed to push. If you are told to resist your body's signals and then told to follow them, it can take some time to get the hang of pushing your baby out.

Speak to your caregiver about how they feel about gentle pushing before complete dilation. Talking about these things before the birth helps everyone to feel in sync during the event.

The Rest and Be Thankful Phase

On the other hand, you may experience the "rest and be thankful" phase (coined by Sheila Kitzinger, famous childbirth educator). You get to 10 centimeters, but don't feel the urge to push. Perhaps the baby isn't low enough to stimulate the Ferguson reflex, which is the bursts of oxytocin that create the urges for pushing. Getting into a more upright position, especially one that opens the pelvis, like squatting, can really move the baby down. Or, maybe your body is just taking a little time to switch over from contractions that dilate to contractions that deliver the baby. That's when you literally rest and be thankful for the break before the hard work of pushing begins.

There are specific tips, tools, and techniques which help during active labor listed in this chapter, but all can be used at any time during labor when you feel it's applicable. Trying positions using the birth ball and practicing techniques during pregnancy will build your comfort in trying them in labor. COMFORT leads to CONFIDENCE which leads to EMPOWERMENT which leads to SUCCESS! We have many clients who feel excited about labor (instead of worried about it) after hearing about the tips and trying the tools and techniques we doulas use to help women cope better.

Tips

Remember the importance of movement, position, relaxation methods, and drawing on your natural resources. The last chapter included tips, tools, and techniques to consider in early labor. We suggest that you expand upon those ideas. Feel free to be creative and develop your skills by choosing new suggestions in this chapter.

For example, when labor intensifies, you may want to continue to use water. Perhaps at home, you took a shower to help labor along. But in active labor, you may need its gate control qualities of making the pain more tolerable, so a bath sounds better. You may have found that resting in a hammock felt right in early labor, but as things intensify, you may want to be up and walking. At home, the classic rock you had on may not work when you arrive at the birth place and feel like nature sounds would be more soothing.

Occasionally, a woman gets out of control, and helping her to get back in control may be required by her partner. Grasp her shoulders (or face), ask her to look at you, and get her to focus on your breathing or vocalization. Then, ask her what she was thinking about during that last contraction and respond to her cues about what might help next time. If she is not sure, offer her a couple of ideas and let her choose.

Rethinking Childbirth Pain

1. Think about the worst pain you have experienced, the flu or a broken leg, surgery, etc. Ask yourself these questions about the pain you felt:

2. How long did it last? – Labor is usually only a half a day.

3. How quickly did the pain peak? – In labor, a woman can adjust to the changing intensity.

4. Was the pain constant? – In labor, built-in breaks allow for rest between contractions.

5. Could you predict when the pain would worsen? – Labor pain has a predictable pattern.

6. What was the reason for your pain? – Labor is pain with a purpose, the physical changes related to progress toward birth.

7. What benefit did you get from your pain? – Birth gives you the reward of your baby.

Tips for Successful Labor

Move and change position – If you move and change position, it can keep labor going and help you stay more comfortable. If you move, the baby can corkscrew its way down and out. Think of how often you change position while sleeping, and then imagine how natural that would be while coping with contractions. We suggest that you change position every half hour or so.

Here are positions you can consider:

* Upright – uses gravity and enhances progress: walking, standing, leaning, kneeling, sitting and slow dancing (Figures 5-10)

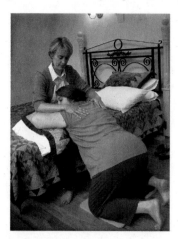

Figure 5. Kneeling and leaning

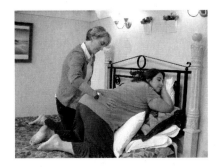

Figure 6. Leaning while being massaged

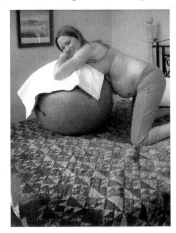

Figure 7. Leaning over the birth ball

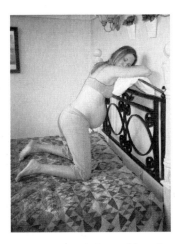

Figure 8. Upright and leaning

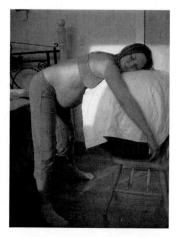

Figure 9. Standing and leaning over the birth ball

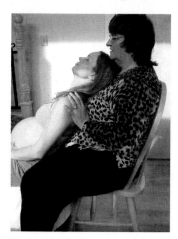

Figure 10. Sitting on ball and leaning back relaxing

- Restful – allows for rest: semi-reclining, reclining and side-lying (Figures 11-13)

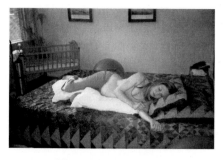

Figure 11. Sidelying

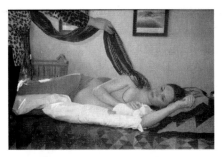

Figure 12. Relaxing with the rebozo

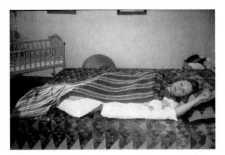

Figure 13. Lying covered with the rebozo

- Squat – opens the pelvis: traditional, modified, stomp, lap, and ball pressed against the wall (Figures 14-18)

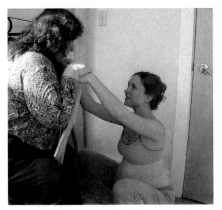

Figure 14. Traditional squat

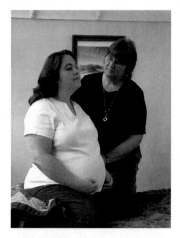

Figure 15. Modified squat

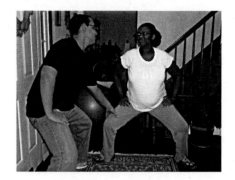

Figure 16. Stomp squat

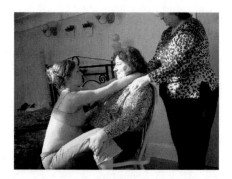

Figure 17. Lap squat

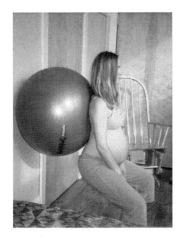

Figure 18. Wall ball squat

- All fours – helps turn a posterior baby: traditional and deep all fours (Figures 19-20)

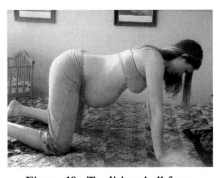

Figure 19. Traditional all fours

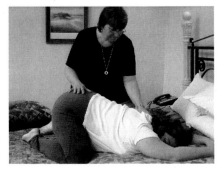

Figure 20. Deep all fours

Here are Examples of How to Use Some Positions to Your Benefit

Slow dancing: Slow dancing in your partner's arms combines many coping strategies: being upright but leaning for support, feeling connected and supported in your partner's arms, swaying back and forth for rhythm, using gate control by having your back massaged, being close to your partner for words of reassurance (Figure 21).

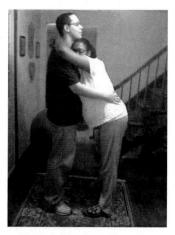

Figure 21. Slow dancing

Side-lying: During Second Stage, you may want to try side-lying for the actual birth. It is comfortable for you, it is easier to curl around the baby to keep it down, your partner can help by supporting your upper leg, and the pressure of the baby's head is not on the perineum, so less tearing usually occurs (Figure 22).

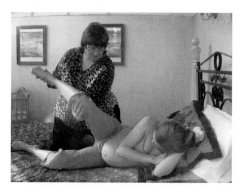

Figure 22. Sidelying - pushing

Lap squat: Maybe you broke your ankle during high school and normal squatting is impossible. In labor, you can sit on your partner's lap, facing him with your arms around his neck and his around your waist (Figure 23). He then opens his knees. This will allow your buttocks to drop between his knees as your legs hook over his. It's a way to open your pelvis without having to support your own body weight. He just closes his knees when the contraction is over and this motion lifts you back onto his lap. Thus the name ... lap squat (Figure 24).

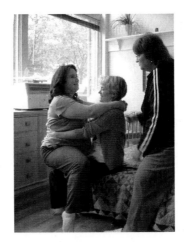

Figure 23. Resting before lap squat

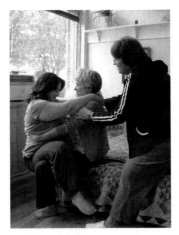

Figure 24. Doing the lap squat

Hands and knees: If the baby is posterior, getting onto your hands and knees can help the baby turn, so labor can progress and your back pain decreases. To save your energy, use the birthing ball (see Figure 7 on page. 81). Kneel on the bed, and then lean over the ball, pressing your breasts and belly onto it. If it feels too hard, place a bed pillow between you and the ball. Hug the ball and turn your head to the side and rest. You can use the ball for pelvic rocking to reduce the pain and your back is available for massage, pressure, warm, cold, vibration, etc.

Relaxation and Breathing – For decades these were the basis of most childbirth classes. More recently, relaxation and other coping skills and tools are being emphasized … since you have been breathing all your life.

How much instruction do you need when you already have years of experience breathing during various situations? For example, how do you breathe while sleeping or trying to relax? Slow and deep. How do you breathe while exercising or when in intense pain? High and light and fast. How do you breathe when you're anxious or scared? First it's high, light, and fast; then it slows and deepens when you feel safe again. You will most likely use all of these ways of breathing, since you will go through all of these things while birthing.

Your birth team's job is to make sure your inhalation equals your exhalation, so you don't hyperventilate. Watch out for dizziness, numbness around your lips, tingling in your fingers—warning signs of hyperventilation. If this happens, cup your hands over your mouth and breathe evenly until the symptoms disappear.

You may find that vocalizing while you breathe can be beneficial, as well. Some women moan (which is good for emotional release) or say positive things (affirmations) or repeat special phrases (rhythm). You can also vocalize through prayer or song. Ask someone to do any of these with you if you desire that kind of support.

When it comes to relaxation, keep these major points in mind:

- **Comfort** – choose a comfortable position and use plenty of pillows for support.

- **Environment** – adjust your surroundings by closing the door, regulating the room temperature, turning off the TV and phone, dimming the lights, playing soothing music and trying your favorite aromatherapy.

- **Breathing** – use slow deep breathing as you would while sleeping to help you relax and to oxygenate you and the baby.

- **Focus** – focus inwardly, with eyes closed to decrease distractions and help you relax.

- **Imagery** – try visualizing a special place where you feel safe, comfortable, and free using your five senses to create it. What would you see, hear, feel, taste and smell if you put yourself in that place?

- **Touch or massage** – communicate to your birth team how and where you want to be touched or massaged.

Tools of the Trade

Labor Bag – Tips for packing your own labor bag are on page 59.

Birthing Ball – A 65-centimeter ball is the suggested size for most women. You will feel the most comfortable and secure if your knees are at right angles when you sit on it (Figure 25). Be sure the ball you use can support your pregnancy weight.

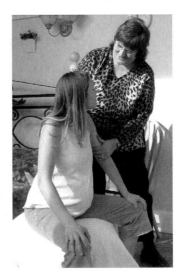

Figure 25. Sitting on the ball

Keep the ball covered for cleanliness and comfort. Tying it in a bed sheet makes it easy to transport. Store the ball away from heat and sharp objects and clean it according to the manufacturer's instructions. You may feel more secure if, while sitting on the ball, you're wedged between two things— for example, your partner and the bed. Leaning forward on a pile of pillows or leaning backwards in your partner's loving arms are great ways to rest while in labor.

During contractions, you can try bouncing, rocking, swaying, or making circles while sitting upright. All these rhythmical movements help align your spine for greater comfort and use gravity to help you make progress. You may want to try writing your name in cursive using the ball during a contraction: having a special task to concentrate on will help you deal with the pain. Sitting on the ball while in the shower is an option, as well. Having water pulsate on your achy back can feel great in labor.

Leaning over the ball while standing or kneeling is a stamina saver. You're getting all the benefits of being upright, but in a more restful position, while the ball absorbs some of your weight. Leaning on the ball against the wall or while in bed gives you support, and you can use rhythm, like gentle bouncing or swaying, to cope.

Cold, warmth, vibration, and massage – You may find one or all of these to be helpful during various phases of labor. Generally, warmth is for mild to moderate pain and cold is for more severe pain. Cool cloths can feel so refreshing and warm blankets can feel so comforting. You can even fill a surgical glove with warm or cold water and tie it like a balloon. Then use it like a hot water bottle or cold compress. You may want to bring a rice sock that can be microwaved or a chemical cold pack that can be activated. And handheld or battery-operated fans are a must!

Vibration can be accomplished by jiggling a hand gently while pressing (against your back for example). Or an actual vibrator can be purchased and used particularly on the back. The vibration causes a local release of endorphins.

Massage techniques are used by many doulas to help you cope better during labor. Sometimes it's to help you to go into a deep relaxed state, and other times it is done in specific areas to help with pain. You guide the doula or your partner by telling them when, where, and how you want it done. The common forms of massage used include effleurage, petrissage, tapotement, and finger glide … plus many variations designed to help you at the time.

Effleurage is massage using long, flowing strokes. The back is an ideal place to do effleurage because of the large body surface. It will tap into the Gate Control Theory of pain relief, since so much skin is being stimulated. Usually, the partner or doula begins at the waist line on your back, since that is a non-threatening place to be touched. You will be very sensitive and may feel vulnerable, so your comfort with any massage is a priority.

A good way to have your partner understand how you would like to be massaged is to reverse roles and show him how and where you prefer it. Plus, he realizes the value of massage, since he's feeling the nice results himself! It can also be done on the arms, legs, and abdomen – your partner will just have to adjust his strength of touch according to the body part or muscle group he's touching. And, you can do it to yourself. Many women find doing a double circular pattern of effleurage on their bellies before labor (and during contractions) feels great.

Petrissage is like kneading, when the muscle is lifted, not pinched. It is most commonly used on tense shoulders. You've probably done this to your partner after a long day at work to relieve shoulder and neck tension. An additional time kneading can be used is during pushing when you may experience a cramp in your legs or buttocks muscles.

Another massage technique great for large muscle cramping or pain is called tapotement (or percussion). They often show this on TV when a masseuse is doing karate chop-like motions on his client. In fact in our doula group, we fondly call it the 'butt chop,' since that's what it is! Try to avoid the boney parts of the body when doing this technique and follow one hand after another.

The last massage technique doulas often use is called a finger glide (or nerve stroke). As the contraction is ending, the massager drags her fingers right down the body part where she began. It signals you that the massage is over. Most massage therapists agree that massage should end where it began.

The critical thing to remember is that you have two jobs and your partner has two jobs. Yours is to communicate and cooperate – communicate what you want and cooperate when touched. The partner's job is to mold his hand to your body part and adjust his strength of touch. That way, he will massage in a way that is both pleasing and beneficial. Practice tensing body parts and letting him touch or massage you to relieve the tension. This is a great way to establish a sensitivity response between the two of you, so you'll automatically release to the touching hand during labor.

There are also many types of massagers you can use: wooden, hard plastic, rolling, frozen, heated, battery, or electric operated. Any form of touch or massage takes advantage of the Gate Control Theory for reducing your pain perception and makes you feel connected to those who are caring for you.

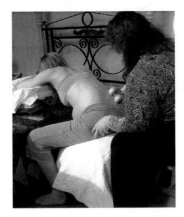

Figure 26. Massage

Acupressure – During pregnancy, massage therapists will avoid certain parts of the expectant woman's body. The hands, feet, and ankles have acupressure points that when stimulated can cause miscarriage. But, during labor, these same points can help enhance progress and ease pain. Two commonly used points are the Hoku Point and Spleen 6 (Figures 27-28). Your partner should press in for a 10 second interval, then release and repeat throughout the contraction.

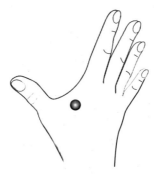

Figure 27. Ho-ku point (where the bones forming the bases of the thumb and index finger come together)

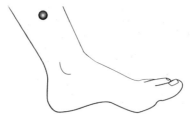

Figure 28. Spleen 6 (4 finger widths above inner aspect of ankle) points

Many women experience trembling during transition or right after birth. To help ease the trembles, try the toe pinch. Grasping a foot with each hand, pinch or press the last three toes firmly and hold (Figure 29). Do this until trembles subside.

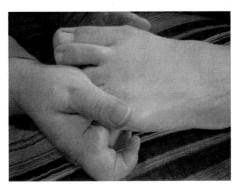

Figure 29. Toe pinch

Hydrotherapy – Many midwives call hydrotherapy their epidural, since women who use it tend to cope better with their pain. A bath not only cleanses you, but often helps to relax you, as well (Gate Control again). A Jacuzzi has the jets to additionally stimulate your skin or provide gentle pressure against an achy back. A shower can affect contractions in a different way: through gravity and nipple stimulation. It can bring on or augment contractions that have slowed or stopped. If the tub or shower isn't available, consider a foot bath, hand bath, or sponge bath. Water in any form seems to be just plain comforting.

When you use water and in what form is something to think about. A bath can slow contractions in early labor (dilutes the oxytocin) or can make them less painful in transition (through Gate Control and relaxation). Since a shower can intensify contractions, you'd want to keep your back to the stream of water during transition, since you wouldn't want to strengthen the contractions any more. The shower can still provide the pain-relief benefits of Gate Control, since so much of your skin is being stimulated.

Pillows – You're probably already using lots of pillows for support and comfort. Many pregnant women use extra pillows: under their head, between their knees while side lying, under their breasts or belly also while side lying, and under their legs or feet for elevation.

Body or pregnancy pillows have become very popular with expectant moms— you may even want to take yours to the birth facility with you. It can be one of your natural comforts, along with other special items you bring from home to make that space yours.

Rebozo – A rebozo is a shawl that some Mexican midwives use during birth. Doulas often carry one in their labor bag. It's a versatile tool. The rebozo can simply cover the mother for warmth or comfort, and aid relaxation (Figure 30). Or it can be used to support various parts of the body for additional relaxation. Birth professionals often use it for assisting with movement or positioning. The rebozo can be used to assist in turning a posterior baby (Figure 31), and it can dramatically help women during pushing. We call this the towel trick (Figure 43).

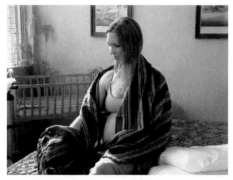

Figure 30. Rebozo wrapped for comfort

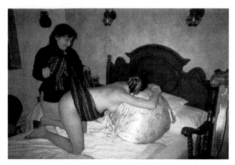

Figure 31. Turning a posterior baby using a rebozo

TENS Device – A TENS device uses transcutaneous electronic nerve stimulation to increase your tolerance to pain. Four electrodes adhere to your back. During a contraction, you power up the device to the level of stimulation that meets your needs. Between contractions, you power it down. Some hospital Physical Therapy departments can rent you one and show you how to use it (Figure 32).

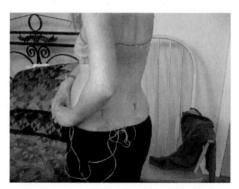

Figure 32. Using the TENS device

Sterile Water Injections – Four injections are done in the Dimples of Venus on your back (right above and to the sides of your tail bone). Sterile water is used to cause a stinging sensation, which your body will respond to by releasing endorphins locally. A midwife or a nurse usually does the procedure. It is not available in all birth facilities.

Doula Techniques

Apron Lift – Women have been using this technique for eons. Place your laced fingers under your belly and lift the baby slowly. Give a little wiggle (sometimes called "shaking the apples") and then put baby back down (Figure 33). Apron lifts can help in several situations: to move a baby back to the center of your belly after sleeping on your side, to lift the engaged baby up for a while near the end of pregnancy, so you can walk around, or to correct an asynclytic baby (bumping its tipped head against the pelvis) during labor. Try having your partner stand behind you and place his hands on your lower belly. Then put your hands on his and help him to do the Apron Lift (Figure 34). Partners seem to really enjoy feeling the baby in this unique way while helping you.

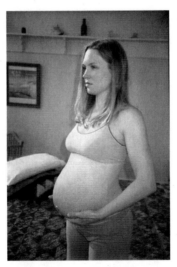

Figure 33. The apron lift

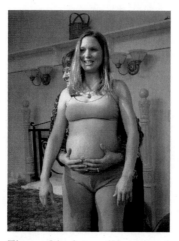

Figure 34. Apron lift assisted

Dangle – This technique elongates your trunk, so a tipped baby's head can possibly right itself. We recommend that the partner puts the ball between his back and the wall and then has you lean your back against his front. Next, he puts his arms forward and you position them under your arms. You both lean against the ball, so it absorbs some of your combined weight, and then you slowly allow yourself to dangle like a limp rag doll, as he supports you with his arms. This can be hard on the partner's back and your underarms. That's why using the ball to support his back is suggested (Figure 35). Consider putting something soft under your arms, as well.

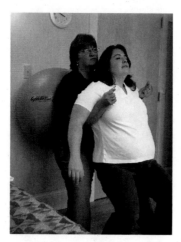

Figure 35. Dangle ball

Counter Pressure – This can help with lower backache in pregnancy or labor. The partner puts the heel of his dominant hand on your tailbone and presses in constantly. Since you may want it done really hard, your partner holds your hip with his free hand, so you don't get pushed forward while he is applying the pressure (Figure 36). Straight counter pressure can be used, or vibration can be added by jiggling the hand. Friction, which causes warmth, can also be applied in a grinding motion while pressing. Both of these variations result in a local release of endorphins.

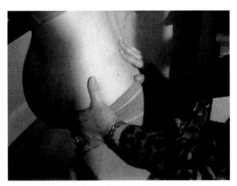

Figure 36. Counterpressure

Lunge – The lunge can be done kneeling or standing. Its purpose is to open up the pelvis in the direction of the lunge. You determine which side of your back hurts and then lunge in that direction. If you're not sure, try both directions. Your body will tell you which is right. If kneeling, one knee is on the bed and the other is at a right angle to your shoulders with your foot resting on the bed. You may find that placing your hand or arm on the upright knee helps you balance (Figure 37). Standing, you do the same, but the foot is on the floor and then the other foot is on the edge of a chair or bed at a right angle. You may enjoy lunging while on the ball (Figure 38). Since you could lose your balance putting your foot up or taking it down, we suggest that the partner spots you by gently holding your waist as you do this type of lunge (Figure 39). You can lunge and hold it for the length of the contraction or go in and out of the lunge…whichever feels better for you.

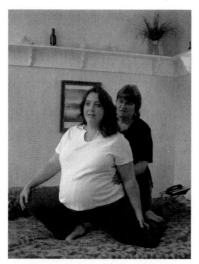

Figure 37. Kneeling lunge

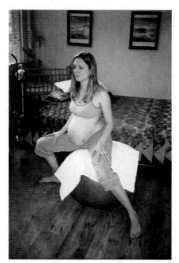

Figure 38. Lunge on the birth ball

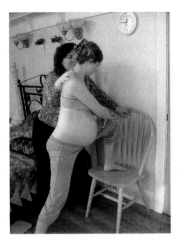

Figure 39. Standing lunge

Knee Press – The knee press helps to tilt your pelvis and decrease the pressure of the baby's head on your nerve endings. You sit in a chair and your partner kneels on one knee in front of you. He puts his hands on the front of your knees and presses towards the back of the chair (Figure 40). This creates a passive pelvic tilt, which helps reduce the pain. He can either rock you back and forth or hold you in the tilt for the whole contraction. The partner can also sit on the floor in front of you and press against your knees using his back to get the same effect—in fact, even stronger (Figure 41)!

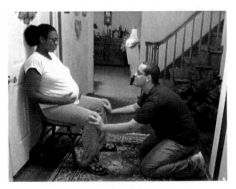

Figure 40. Hand knee press

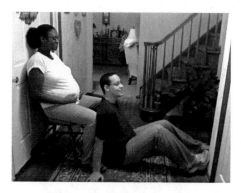

Figure 41. Back knee press

Hip Squeeze and the Double Hip Squeeze – The hip squeeze opens the hips much like squatting does, but someone does it for you. You lean over while someone presses in diagonally on both sides of your outer hips, so the pelvic outlet increases in size. *Be sure they do not push in and up or the outlet will become smaller.* Doing the double hip squeeze using two people (one on each side of the hips) can really make a difference because of the added strength behind the squeezing (Figure 42).

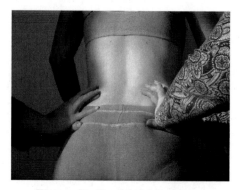

Figure 42. Double hip squeeze

The Doula Hula – The doula hula is when you get on all fours on the floor and the doula straddles your hips with her knees, as she stands above you. She then presses her knees together, which squeezes your hips, while she rotates them in a circular motion. The combined techniques can assist the baby to adjust itself more easily, due to the increased space and the actual movement.

So you probably feel more ready to deal with whatever comes your way after filling your brain (and labor bag) with all these tips, tools, and techniques. Knowledge is empowering and knowing what to use and when can really make all the difference. Remember to encourage your birth team to think outside the box—

they should be creative, constantly brainstorm ideas, and use problem solving whenever it's needed. Our clients often tell us that what they appreciated the most was how intuitive we were in knowing what the mother needed, even before she communicated it herself—or even thought of it. But that's just the power of knowledge and experience. You may not be able to have the experience, but you can arm yourself with knowledge. You'll feel empowered by the knowledge and skills you developed, which will help you to stay confident about your ability to do this awesome task. Millions of women before you drew on their inner wisdom and natural resources to give birth – **you can do it, too**!

Chapter 7
Birthing the Baby

Scenario 1: Pushing in an Unmedicated Labor

Jeri was having her first baby. Her labor was in its seventh hour and the last few minutes had been the most challenging. She felt like she couldn't go on. She felt tired, nauseous, and had cold shivers. She wondered how much longer it would be.

Suddenly, she arched her back: "I'm feeling pressure, a lot of pressure!" she said.

As her midwife got ready to check her cervix, Jeri broke in moaning: "I'm pushing."

Her midwife told her to pant, while she quickly checked her cervix. "You are completely dilated," she said. "You can start pushing when you want to."

Jeri and her husband were so relieved; they had been waiting for this moment. With the next contraction, Jeri felt the urge to bear down build and as she pushed, she felt her baby moving down. She curled around her baby and pushed with each contraction.

Soon her midwife took Jeri's hand and placed it on her baby's head. "Your baby is crowning—this is your baby's head," she said. Although Jeri was tired, feeling her baby suddenly made it all seem real to her. She pushed again and her baby's head slipped out.

Soon, the rest of the body was born. "You have a baby girl!" her midwife said.

Scenario 2: Pushing with an Epidural

Georgia had been in labor for hours and hours. She had gotten an epidural at 5 cm dilation because she needed the rest. It was very late at night, so Georgia and her husband slept after the epidural was given.

In the morning, her doctor came to check on her and found that her cervix was completely effaced and dilated. "You can start pushing now, or we can turn down the epidural and give you time to labor down," her doctor told Georgia.

Georgia couldn't move her legs very much because they were so heavy from the medication. So she asked to have the epidural turned down. Georgia waited for her legs to feel stronger and to feel rectal pressure that did not go away between contractions.

In two hours, she felt strong rectal pressure. Her doctor checked her again and discovered that the baby's head was at plus two station in her pelvis. "Let's start pushing now," her doctor suggested.

Georgia's husband had her take a deep cleansing breath and blow it out, and then told her to take another breath and hold it while he counted to ten. The nurse encouraged her, shouting "Push, push, push, push, as hard as you can!"

Georgia held her breath and pushed three times during each contraction. It went slowly. She pushed and rested and pushed and rested. It took several tries before she started to push in the right place to move the baby down.

"Georgia, that's the right push," her doctor encouraged her. "Do another one just like that one."

The nurse and her husband kept shouting, "Good! Push, push, harder! Harder!"

After an hour, the doctor had the nurse get the room ready for the baby's birth. The large light came down to shine on her perineum. The mini-surgical table was in place in case she needed stitches. The doctor put the bed up very high, so that the baby's crowning head would be at the doctor's eye level.

Georgia was semi-sitting, with her legs pulled back toward her as far as they would go. She pushed and pushed and her face became purple with her efforts. Forty minutes later, her baby boy was born, and her proud husband cut the cord.

Pushing Feels Different

There are two main types of work involved in having a baby. The first type is relaxing into the contractions to allow your cervix to open and to let the baby come down into your birth canal. That's the first stage of labor. This chapter is about the second stage of labor, which is the pushing part. Once your cervix has been checked and you've found out that you're 100% effaced and 10 cm dilated, you'll be able to start pushing your baby out—if you feel the urge to push. You might not be feeling the urge to push yet, although your cervix is complete. Your baby's head may not be down low enough to stimulate the bundle of nerves that produces the urge to push.

Although second stage is the most instinctive part of birth, the sensations vary from woman to woman. The urge to push feels very different from earlier contractions. Many women who disliked the work involved in first stage—relaxing into the contractions—find they really enjoy pushing. You can finally do something to give birth, aside from tolerating the pain of dilation. You may have heard many descriptions of second stage that ranged from scary to strange to enjoyable. Many women, especially those who do not have an epidural, find second stage very relieving. Keep in mind that most babies will fit very well through the birth canal, and that even large babies are not ten pounds of head. And of course, right after the work of pushing, you get to greet your baby. This is what all the work is about!

If this is your first baby, keep in mind that pushing may take longer for this birth than in future births. Be prepared to pace yourself. The contractions usually space themselves further apart (approximately every five minutes) and you will be able to push, then take a break. Be sure to really rest between pushes.

There are three distinct parts to the pushing stage, just as there were in labor. These are early, active, and transition. The early part is the rest-and-be-thankful phase (that's what Sheila Kitzinger, a famous childbirth educator, calls it). Not every woman will experience this as a separate part. You get to 10 centimeters, but don't feel the urge to push. Perhaps the baby isn't low enough to stimulate the Ferguson reflex (bursts of oxytocin that create the urge to push). Getting into a more upright position, especially one that opens the pelvis, like squatting, can really move the baby down. Or maybe your body is just taking a little time to switch over from contractions that dilate to contractions that deliver the baby. That's when you literally rest and be thankful for the break before the hard work of pushing begins.

In the active phase, the baby's head will play peek-a-boo as it descends, coming lower during your pushes, and then sneaking back up a little bit after pushing. This continues until your baby's head moves past the pubic bone and is lying directly on the perineum.

Throughout pushing, feel free to try whatever position feels comfortable to you. Although most hospitals routinely have mothers in a semi-reclining position, many women prefer to be side-lying. Other women enjoy the hands-and-knees position or kneeling and leaning against the upright head of the bed. Side-lying and hands and knees are positions encouraged by midwives because the pressure of the baby's head is not against the perineum. This means fewer tears.

Some women enjoy standing, squatting, or sitting on the toilet or a birthing chair. Most women don't enjoy pushing while flat on their backs. Try out various positions at home and think about bearing down. (Never actually bear down while pregnant if your cervix is not fully dilated, as this can cause tenderness to your cervix.) Think about what positions are comfortable and feel normal to you. For instance, if you are instructed to pull your knees to your ears and that doesn't feel right, you could place the soles of your feet together instead.

The third phase of pushing is when the baby is crowning and the head is about to be born. We call this the transitional phase because it is emotionally and physically intense for you. The key to this part of pushing is to go slow and steady. You don't want to rush here. You want to give your perineum a chance to stretch and blossom out. You should use warm compresses and have gentle support on your perineum as the baby's head crowns.

At this time, your caregivers will probably want you to be in a position that they feel comfortable catching the baby in. Babies can be wet and slippery at birth! It's also a good idea to ask your caregiver about what positions you can use during pushing. Some caregivers are open to whatever you are comfortable with. Others are less open to certain positions.

How Gravity Can Help

Upright positions can help you throughout pushing. If you are upright, gravity will assist your pushes to bring the baby closer. If you are in the lithotomy position (the stirrups position) or the semi-lithotomy position (stirrups but slightly sitting up), your pelvis is tilted back and you will be pushing your baby's head uphill. That will make your work harder! Also, if the baby's head is crowning and you are in the lithotomy position, the weight of gravity will bring more pressure from the baby's head onto your perineum, and you will be more likely to tear. A more upright position will have the head exert more even pressure all around your vaginal opening. Even pressure will help you stretch instead of tear.

Upright positions, like squatting or standing, will speed up the descent of the baby's head. Squatting also enlarges the pelvis, shortens the birth canal, and uses gravity very well to bring the baby's head down quickly. If you are a gardener or have good squatting muscles from yoga or other exercises, you may like this position. But during crowning, squatting may be *too* upright. You want to allow time for your perineum to stretch, so you don't tear. This may be a good time to switch to side-lying or kneeling and leaning your head and arms over the back of the bed. Those positions are less upright than squatting.

The Support You Need Now

During pushing, you'll need to have cold compresses ready for your forehead, a fan, and something cool to drink (or ice chips). You may need someone to help hold your legs or remind you to get in a more comfortable position. You will also enjoy warm compresses for your perineum. They help with stretching and help you feel where to push (the warmth helps guide your pushing). You may need someone to help direct your pushing—although pushing the way your body wants to push (see "How to Work with Nature" below) is preferable. You may also need encouragement and loving support during the hard work. Your partner or doula can help you by reminding you to "ease your baby out" and "bring your baby down."

Some nurses will describe pushing as feeling "like a really big bowel movement." They say this because the pressure of the baby's head is stimulating the nerve endings which signal the urge to have a bowel movement. But that's not the image that you as a birthing mother will want to be left with. If your nurse says that, then your partner should counter this image with a more appropriate one, such as "bulge your bottom" or "you can feel the baby coming."

Should You Take Birthing Photos?

Should you have a support person take labor and birthing photos? We're in favor of it. First-time moms often feel that crowning and other intimate photos of birth are not necessary. This is, of course, your own preference. But we have heard moms who did not have these pictures wonder what they would have been like. Unless you have a mirror positioned in the right place and you can concentrate enough during pushing to look into the mirror, you won't see your baby emerge. Your eyes are on the side opposite the belly. After your beautiful baby is born, you'll wonder how he could have ever fit inside you. Could you really have given birth to him?

Most women are very interested in their birth pictures. If you don't want to look at them, tuck them in a drawer for a while; maybe you'll look at them months later. You can even throw them away if you don't want them. But you can't put the baby back in and say, "Action!" There are no do-overs.

Another helpful hint: Your due date is just an estimate. Consider carrying a disposable camera in your purse from week 35 on. If your baby comes unexpectedly early, you can still have photos. A nurse or doctor can always take pictures with your camera if you can't take them.

Caregiver Discussion Questions

Have a frank discussion with your caregiver about second stage and how he or she usually handles catching the baby if everything is going well. Will he support your perineum with warm compresses? What positions will he allow? How often does he do episiotomies? Under what circumstances does he do them? What does he do differently if meconium is present? Will your partner be able to cut the cord (if he wishes)?

If you are giving birth in a hospital, does your doctor always break the bed apart? Does your doctor attend all of second stage or is he in and out until the baby's head is crowning? Some doctors will watch a push or two in the first part of pushing and then decide how long they think it will take and leave for a while. If you don't have a doula to help you, you and your partner may be alone for a while or just have a nurse present.

How to Work with Nature

If you feel the strong urge to push, your body will naturally start pushing. Get into the position you feel comfortable pushing in and push the way your body wants to push. This is called *physiologic* pushing.

While you're pushing, you'll continue to breathe. You may feel like grunting or moaning. Deep guttural sounds mean you are working. High pitched sounds mean you are afraid. Most women prefer not to hold their breath. Some women will hold their breath for short periods of about five seconds. To help pushing along, curl around your baby as you push. Try not to take a huge breath in while you are pushing during a contraction. Each huge inhalation will raise your diaphragm and pull your baby's head back up a bit. Instead, as you continue to push, curl forward around your baby in one steady motion, taking small breaths whenever you need to. This helps keep the peek-a-boo of your baby's head coming lower, then going back up, to a minimum.

Purple pushing is another term for medical pushing. This is the type of pushing where you take a couple of deep breaths and let them out. On the third inhalation, you take another huge breath (as if you are going deep under water) and then hold it while someone counts to ten—fairly slowly. You repeat this three or more times per contraction. By the end of the contraction, your face is purple and you need to breathe very deeply because you and your baby are now short of oxygen. If you want to see purple pushing in action, ask your partner to hold his breath while you count. See if he turns purple. He'll be convinced it's not for you!

Women often have to take a contraction off after medical pushing to allow the baby's heart rate to recover. What does it say to you when a maneuver is encouraged that can cause your baby stress? Sometimes during purple pushing the mom may need to wear an oxygen mask because her baby's heart rate goes down and she needs to send more oxygen to her baby. An extended period of purple pushing can lead to broken capillaries in and around the mom's eyes. It can also lead to hemorrhoids or worsen the ones you already have. Taking a deep breath and pushing hard, and then taking another deep breath also adds to perineal tearing, because the baby's head becomes like a battering ram against the mom's pelvic floor. On the other hand, slow sustained pushing, like physiologic pushing, brings the baby down in one sustained rocking motion, helping the perineum to blossom out slowly.

The best time to use directed pushing is if you have an epidural and are not feeling enough sensations to push without directed help. Even if you do have an epidural, try turning it down first and doing physiologic pushing. If this works for you, you will have a gentler delivery. However, if pushing becomes lengthy and you become exhausted, you will have a greater chance of having an assisted delivery, either by instruments or cesarean birth.

Poor Dr. Valsalva

Medical pushing was conceived when obstetricians chose to combine doing episiotomies with the Valsalva maneuver. They surmised that this approach would get the babies out faster. The Valsalva maneuver was invented by Dr. Antonio Maria Valsalva, a 17th century Italian doctor, for clearing the inner ear. It was never intended for use during birth, especially when head compressions are already reducing oxygen flow to the baby. Poor Dr. Valsalva would likely be dismayed at the use we are making of his little maneuver.

But because so many women choose to have epidurals and can't feel the urges to bear down, medical pushing has remained in use. Since *directed* pushing can either be the physiologic approach or the medical approach, which way makes more sense to you to try?

How to Avoid *Unnecessary* Interventions

If you can avoid getting an epidural, you will make pushing much easier for yourself. Epidurals *do* help you relax during the cervical dilation part of labor, but they can make it much harder to coordinate your efforts when you are pushing.

Upright positions and changing positions also help avoid assisted deliveries because gravity is working in your favor. Also, having a doula helps you avoid vacuum or forceps assistance because she knows techniques to try during pushing. For instance, you can use the towel trick (Figure 43). The towel trick involves the mother holding one end of a long towel or rebozo that has been knotted at each end. The doula or partner holds the other end. During pushing, you do a tug of war which encourages the mother to get into a "C" shape around the baby. This helps to keep the baby's head from slipping back up between pushes. This also gives the mother something else to pull on other than her legs, which many women find uncomfortable.

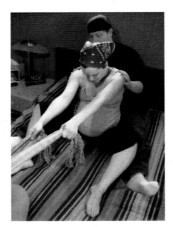

Figure 43. Towel trick using a rebozo

What Is Laboring Down?

If your cervix is completely effaced and dilated, you can begin pushing. If you don't feel the urge to push you should just rest and be thankful. This is what we call *laboring down or passive descent*. There is no need to push until the baby is low enough to activate the nerves that give you the urge to push usually at around plus 1 or plus 2 station. Your contractions will continue to bring the baby down lower without you actively pushing. That is the essence of laboring down.

If you have an epidural in place, laboring down may also include turning the epidural medication down or off, so that you will be able to feel the urge to push as much as possible.

Just What Is the Perineum?

The perineum is the region between the vagina and the anus. It is a central structure in the pelvic floor. It includes the perineal membrane and is also the point of insertion for eight different pelvic floor muscles (Figure 44). These muscles help support your inner organs, such as the uterus, bladder and rectum. So it's a very important area, especially during birth.

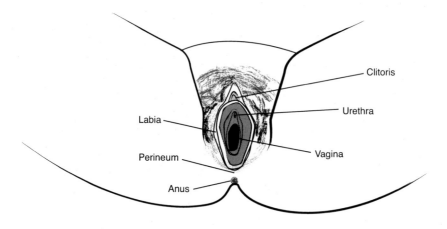

Figure 44. External female anatomy

Why Avoid an Episiotomy?

An episiotomy is a surgical incision (cut) of the perineum to enlarge the vaginal opening during birth. Most women would prefer to avoid having an episiotomy unless the health of the baby makes a fast delivery necessary. Talk to your doctor or midwife. How often are episiotomies done in their practice? If your caregiver is an obstetrician, he is also a surgeon, and may have strong feelings about whether it is easier to repair a tear or an incision. Check to see how your doctor feels. You may also want to discuss other methods your doctor may use during pushing, like manual enlargement of the vagina. It can encourage tearing or the need for an episiotomy.

You probably will prefer to spontaneously separate (tear), rather than have an episiotomy. A separation often involves just the skin; an episiotomy is through the muscle. Even the smallest episiotomy is longer and deeper than most tears. So there is more blood loss, risk of infection, and increased pain after childbirth. Women who have had an episiotomy tend to postpone sexual relations far longer than women who don't. You probably want to choose a doctor who has a low episiotomy rate.

For several weeks before your due date, have your partner help you do perineal massage every evening (see "Prenatal Perineal Massage"). The massage will help your tissues stretch and loosen. It also helps to prepare you for the burning and stretching sensations of crowning.

Midwives Support the Perineum

Midwives practice so that tears and episiotomies are rare. Instead, they use warm compresses, physiologic pushing, lubricant, and full support of the vaginal opening during crowning. This helps the baby's head slip out through a blossoming perineum. This greatly reduces tearing. It also helps for you to push slowly when the baby's head is crowning. Usually, the midwife will help direct you to breathe or pant while your baby's head and shoulders are born. She may apply firm pressure on your perineum while using warm compresses or lubricant, and she will give you time to open as you were meant to (Figure 45).

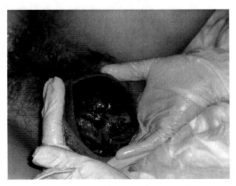

Figure 45. Supporting the perineum during crowning

Here are some ways to avoid perineal tearing:

- Concentrate on good nutrition.

- Do Kegel exercises.

- Take vitamins C and E and bioflavonoids to improve skin elasticity.

- Practice the "open position" during pregnancy, as described in Francoise Barbira Freedman's *Yoga for Pregnancy*: Kneel on both knees with buttocks resting on heels and palms on the floor in front of you. Lift your left knee, so it is beside your left arm, with your left foot flat on the floor. Your left hip is raised slightly higher than the right. The right buttock rests on the right foot. Switch sides. This opens the base of the body as widely as possible, so the muscles are pre-stretched before birth.

Prenatal Perineal Massage:

- Sit in a comfortable position. Use a lubricant, like extra virgin olive oil, and work it into the vagina, perineum, and labia. This is easier to do if you are sitting upright.

- Place your thumbs just inside the vagina and your index fingers just outside the vagina, so the perineum is in between. If your partner helps, lie down and he will insert index fingers and use thumbs on the outside.

- Massage in a U shape back and forth from center. Rub the skin with just enough pressure, so you feel a slight stinging sensation. Release as you feel the pressure and stinging. Guide your partner if he is helping you.

- As you progress, you will notice more elasticity before stinging occurs. Skip a day or two if you have pain or swelling afterwards.

- Keep in mind, this is not recommended if you have active herpes or a vaginal infection, or if the massages cause swelling.

An Epidural Splits the Mind and the Body

Pushing is more difficult with an epidural in place than if you are unmedicated. It's also true that having an epidural usually lengthens the time that you will spend pushing your baby out. Having an epidural increases your chances of needing an assisted delivery. If you push for more than three hours or your baby's heart rate goes down after so much purple pushing, you may need to have a vacuum or forceps delivery, or even a cesarean birth.

Why is it harder to push with an epidural? The epidural creates a mind/body split. You can't feel your body's messages about how and where to push. Mothers who have experienced birth with an epidural and birth without one talk about how pushing feels completely different in each one. With an epidural, you can just barely feel that you are having a contraction, and so you start to push. You try to push where you think the baby's head is, but it is more a mental exercise of imagining where to push.

When your labor is unmedicated, you usually feel strong pressure that builds until you do what you need to do—and that is pushing your baby out and giving birth. You don't need much coaching because your body, like the bodies of other mothers throughout the ages, does what comes naturally. You work with your body. You follow your body's messages. You don't have to think about it or imagine what to do—it's instinctive. The next thing you know your baby is born!

Chapter 8

Right after the Birth

The sound of a baby's cries rang out in the birth center. The baby had just been born, and the midwife helped June place her daughter onto her chest while she wiped the baby and made sure the baby was breathing and looked fine. Mark had tears in his eyes as he beheld his daughter for the first time. Soon, the baby's cord stopped pulsing and the midwife helped Mark cut the cord. While June held her daughter, they waited a few minutes until the midwife asked her to give a few small pushes, and she easily delivered the placenta. A nurse finished wiping off the baby while June held her, and then she placed warm blankets over both of them.

June's legs were trembling, so her doula pinched her toes—a little trick that often helps get rid of the shakes. Then her doula helped June get her new daughter to her breast. While the baby sniffed around and started to try to latch on, Mark and June were looking at their daughter. They decided that they would call her Ariel.

June's doula brought her some juice to drink and asked her if she wanted to have some hot tea. Meanwhile, the doula and Mark took the first family pictures. June's midwife carefully checked her perineum and birth canal for tears that might need stitches, but she didn't need any. The midwife also checked to make sure that June wasn't bleeding too heavily and that she and the baby were comfortable. June hadn't even realized that her midwife had given Ariel Apgar scores of 9 and 9 while she was holding her.

June iced the cake she had made earlier and put "Happy Birthday Ariel" on it. She passed out cake to everyone to celebrate the birth.

June relaxed and nursed and held Ariel. Her doula brought June and Mark a breakfast of scrambled eggs and toast. When June was ready to relax, her midwife weighed Ariel, measured her, and diapered her. Then June, Ariel, and Mark had their first of many naps together.

What to Expect the First Two Hours

Those first moments right after the birth are very important for establishing a relationship with your baby. The baby will enter a period called the quiet alert state.

During this time you will want to get to know your baby, bond with your baby, and initiate breastfeeding. But before you start to envision how your new family will bond, keep in mind that where you give birth and who your caregivers are will make a difference as to how the immediate postpartum period will go.

Your baby has been born and takes his first breath in the new world, and you have choices to make about cutting the cord. Some mothers like to postpone cutting the cord for a brief time to allow the cord to stop pulsating. This allows the baby to get any residual oxygen, hormones, and nutrients from the placenta. Others choose to have the cord cut right away. If you are doing cord-blood collection, the caregiver can wait until the cord has stopped pulsing. Another decision about the cord is who cuts it. Sometimes moms do it, sometimes dads do it, and sometimes the caregiver or doula cuts the cord.

After the baby is born and the cord is cut, you still need to deliver your baby's placenta (Figure 46). This is an easy process compared to the birth of the baby, since it weighs about 1/6 of the baby's weight. You may need to push a little, about ten minutes or so after your baby is born, to deliver the placenta. Your caregiver will need to make certain that the placenta is intact, that there are not pieces of it left in your uterus (Figure 47). Then your caregiver will need to look closely at your vagina and perineum to see if tearing occurred and whether you will need repair stitches.

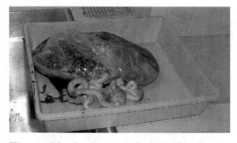

Figure 46. A placenta, baby's first home

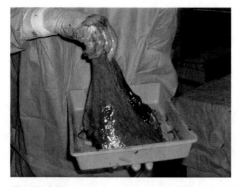

Figure 47. Holding up the sac attached to the placenta

Meanwhile, staff will be assessing the health of your newborn. They will make sure your baby's breathing and heart rate are good and then assign *Apgar scores*. This assessment can be done right next to you or the baby could be on your chest. In a hospital, it is typical for the baby to be taken to a warmer, often in your labor room, for these assessments. Your partner can go with the baby and talk to her or take photos. But you should find out how your caregiver normally handles this time immediately after your baby's birth, so you will be prepared and not have any surprises.

Table 5. Apgar Scores

A score is taken at 1 minute and 5 minutes after birth. This is a very general test to see how the newborn is responding after birth. Typically, the score will be given as two numbers, for example: 8, 9, meaning an 8 at 1 minute after birth and a 9 at five minutes. Ten is possible, but almost no tens are given.

They look for:	0 points	1 point	2 points
Activity—muscle tone	floppy or absent	flexing of arms and legs	active movement
Pulse	absent	below 100 bpm	above 100 bpm
Grimace	no response	grimace	sneezes, pulls away
Appearance of skin color	blue, grey, pale	normal except extremities	all over normal
Respiration	absent	slow, regular	good crying

Meanwhile, you have just given birth, so you will be *in recovery* for about two hours. Your vitals will be monitored. Your uterus will be palpated or massaged every few minutes to make sure it is firm and you are not bleeding too much. This palpation is usually uncomfortable, so using slow, deep breathing can help. Ask the nurse to show you how to massage your own uterus. You'll probably do it more frequently and more gently. While the nurse is massaging, a good distraction for you is to be holding your baby, or if that is not yet possible, to have your partner hold your baby near you. After all, you've been longing to see her for months.

Choices about Baby Care

If you have had a vaginal birth, many states require that the baby be given an antibiotic eye ointment to prevent certain infections to which the baby might have been exposed while passing through the vaginal canal. Early in pregnancy, you were tested for STDs. These STDs can lead to blindness in babies if not treated. The eye ointment can be postponed until after your first bonding and nursing. The ointment will blur the baby's vision, which could interfere with your early bonding experience. Some parents choose to waive the ointment altogether. If this appeals to you, talk to your care provider about how to do it.

A vitamin K shot, which promotes the clotting factor, is also routinely given to the baby after birth. You can waive or postpone this, if you wish. Your baby's body will establish its own clotting factor within eight days after birth. The clotting factor is especially important if you plan to have your boy circumcised. It is also advised if your baby needs any surgery or sometimes for forehead bruising (to reduce the spread of the bruise).

Another choice you can make is to ask to be fully informed of any tests—and the reasons for the tests—that the caregivers wish to do to your baby. Remember, this is *your* baby. You are now parents and decision makers. Your doctors should be able to explain clearly why they wish to take a blood sample or check your baby's blood sugar, for example. You may wish to put into your birth vision that your baby is never to go to the nursery or be out of your sight without the presence of one of her parents. It is always good to be informed about any procedure, even if you don't object to any test your doctor suggests.

Newborn Appearance

Your newborn will be the most beautiful baby ever born! But you might have some questions about some of the things you see on her, especially if this is your first baby.

Vernix is the waxy yellow-white coating that protected her skin while she lived in her liquid environment inside you. She may have *milia* or little white pimple-like bumps on her face. They are just blocked pores and will clear soon. You will notice that her head looks bigger in proportion to her body than yours does as an adult. Your baby's head might also be cone-shaped for a few hours after birth from molding during her passage through the birth canal.

You might be interested in counting your baby's fingers and toes as soon as she is born, and seeing what color her hair is. Many hospitals will immediately wrap your infant up, like a baby burrito, to make sure she stays warm. They will also give her a cap to wear, so that she doesn't lose too much body heat from her head. You may unwrap her to look at her, but take care to wrap her back up soon or keep her skin-to-skin with you.

Your baby may have a *birth mark* on her forehead (sometimes called angel kisses) or on the back of her neck called a stork bite. These marks are blotchy pinkish and are the most common form of birthmark (about 70%). Some darker skinned babies can have birth marks called Mongolian spots. Your baby's doctor will show you any birth marks your baby has and tell you whether they will need any treatment (most often they don't).

Lanugo is the dark hair that some babies have on their body that drops off in about a week. The hair on your newborn's head may also change. Your baby could be born with dark hair, which is replaced later by light hair. Most babies' eyes look slate blue when born. They can actually see best from mother's nipple line to her face. Their final eye color sets in several months later. Your baby's eyes may cross once in awhile. That is normal, too.

She will be born with dozens of reflexes and responses. It is so much fun discovering them as she does her first yawn, sneeze, or smile. And no, smiling does not mean *gas*! It's amazing to see how your baby will change over the next weeks and months.

Some great photo ops
Try to get these pictures:

- Midwife or doctor handing the baby to mom for skin-to-skin bonding

- The cord being cut

- Baby being foot-printed and weighed

- Nude baby picture (for future prom-date embarrassment)

- First diaper

- First nursing with partner looking on

- Dad holding baby

- Family picture

- Family picture with doctor or midwife

- Family picture with doula

- Grandparents with baby, siblings with baby

- Baby's first home—the placenta (ask doctor or midwife to open up the sac to show you where the baby was)

Caring for Yourself Right after Birth

Even if you've labored for a long time and felt exhausted just before your wonderful baby was born, you'll probably experience a second wind of energy after he's born. You'll be excited to meet and hold your baby as soon as possible. In fact, holding or seeing your baby up close will help you begin your recovery. This is what you've been waiting so long for.

You shouldn't think of your baby as separate from yourself. You should expect to be treated as a unit. Physically and emotionally, you will need your baby near you, just as your baby will need you. Unless there is some specific medical necessity, let your caregivers know ahead of time that you do not want to be separated postpartum. Be sure to request rooming-in, so that you can maintain the closeness that is so important for bonding. Partners often spend the first night or longer with mom and baby, so that the mom can get rest and do rooming-in.

As soon as you can, get something to eat and drink. You should have a balanced meal that includes protein, carbohydrates, and fat. You've just done a big job, and you need to replenish yourself. Remember to keep well hydrated, since fluids are so important for the nursing mother.

You may need an icepack to take care of any vaginal swelling or irritation from the birth. The staff will offer you several other remedies, such as using a peri-bottle while urinating, sitting in a sitz bath to encourage healing, and using analgesic creams for the discomfort. They'll suggest that you blot, not wipe, from front to back. If you have hemorrhoids, they'll provide witch-hazel pads, stool softeners, and maybe cortisone suppositories. Your caregiver will also instruct you about how and when to take sitz baths.

Time Alone as a New Family

You may have relatives who are longing to see you and meet your new baby. First, take the time to get cleaned up and fed, and to breastfeed your baby. Organize yourself. Many couples choose not to call their family until after the birth. This helps take some of the pressure off. If your family is already waiting at your birth place, postpone seeing them until after you've had quiet time to bond with just the three of you. You're not ready to be a hostess yet.

Your First Breastfeeding

Try to get your baby to the breast within the first half-hour to hour after his birth. During his early quiet and alert time, just after birth, your baby will likely be very open to trying his first nursing. Bring your baby to your breast as his mouth opens very wide, like a baby bird. Latch him onto as much of the areola beyond the nipple as he can. Your baby will have an instinct to nurse. Get help if you need it. But don't worry! Your baby isn't starving. Allow him to explore around your breast. See how he does. If you give him skin-to-skin contact and he just nuzzles and smells your breasts, that's okay. Try expressing some of your colostrum onto your nipple for him to taste. This will help give him the idea of where the food comes from.

When your baby has latched on and begins to suck, you'll feel a deep tugging sensation. You'll be able to see his cheeks move and see him sucking. With a strong latch, your baby's suck will keep him on the breast. If your baby's mouth keeps coming off of your breast, keep working to improve his latch. But remember, with this first nursing, enjoy! Don't allow it to become stressful. You can always try again a little later.

Newborn Reflexes

Your baby is born with several reflex responses that will help him to adjust to postpartum life. The most important ones are to breathe, suck, and swallow. Some other interesting reflexes include:

- **The rooting reflex:** If you tickle your baby's cheek, you will stimulate the rooting reflex, in which he opens his mouth and turns his head, searching for the breast.

- **The startle reflex:** When your baby is moved unexpectedly or quickly or his arms encounter something strange, he will throw up his arms and tremble.

- **The hand gripping reflex:** Babies are born with a strong grasp and will be able to grip your finger tightly. Dads love this one!

- **The stepping reflex:** When you stand a newborn upright, he will make stepping motions.

- **The crawling position:** Watch your newborn as you place him on his tummy. He will move into what looks like a crawling position. Your newborn is amazing!

Now You'll Want to Spread the News

After you've given yourself time to bond with your baby, you'll be eager to spread your joyous news. But you may have just given birth in the middle of the night, so know your audience. Some of your family and friends will want the news in the morning. But be mindful of your own needs, too. If you haven't slept in a while, you may want to ask your close relatives to let you rest before they visit you and see the baby. You'll have taken plenty of pictures to share with them, even if they meet your baby half a day after the birth. Introduce siblings gently. Think about keeping your first child's routine going. Most hospitals and birth centers offer tours or classes for siblings to better understand what is about to happen. It's a nice way to include them in the pregnancy and birth.

If you do have visitors, keep them to a minimum and keep visits short. If someone is going to help and support you, that's great. You know which of your relatives will deplete your energy and which ones will help you recover. Now and in the following days and weeks, ask the ones who are truly helpful to give you the support you need. Gently tell the ones who deplete you that you can only have short visits because you are recovering.

Chapter 9

Cesarean Birth and Vaginal Birth after Cesarean

Sheila had decided to have a homebirth with midwives. But as the pregnancy progressed, tests showed that Sheila had gestational diabetes. That placed her in the high-risk group, which meant her care was transferred to perinatologists. It also meant a hospital birth.

As Sheila got closer to her due date, the baby turned into a breech position. She tried natural techniques to turn the baby, but none worked for her. The doctor decided to try an external version, but the position of the cord made it impossible.

So they set up a scheduled cesarean according to when he was available, since he was her favorite doctor.

Sheila and her husband had a doula attend the birth, even though it was a scheduled cesarean delivery. They had developed a touch-and-trust relationship with their doula, so it only seemed natural to have her attend. They knew they could count on her to guide them through their highly medicalized birth. And the parents-to-be felt very reassured when they saw the doula's personal and professional relationship with the staff.

The doula kept them calm through music, massage, and tender words before the birth. She informed them about what to expect, so there would be no surprises during surgery. She stayed with Sheila from her gowning up upon arrival, through the cesarean birth, and well into their bonding and nursing afterwards. The doula took birth and newborn pictures to document their special event.

Everyone who saw the birth agreed that it had certainly been a family-centered cesarean birth. So even though it wasn't what Sheila had originally envisioned, her birth really did turn out to be woman-centered. And wonderful baby boy Simon was her reward at the end!

Call It a Cesarean Birth

There's a lot you can do to avoid the major surgery of a cesarean birth. But sometimes a cesarean birth is necessary. You can still have a wonderful family-centered birth. And you can still have a vaginal birth after you've had a cesarean.

Why do we call it a cesarean *birth,* rather than a cesarean section or C-section? A cesarean birth is still *your* birth, and the birth of your child. If you've given birth via cesarean, it helps you to heal afterwards if you can focus on the birth of your child, rather than on the surgery. Even if you've had a cesarean, you've still given birth to your child. Just think of it as it an alternate birth route!

Avoid It if You Can

A cesarean birth, even if it is scheduled, will be far harder on your body than almost any vaginal birth would be. Your first effort should be to avoid a cesarean birth as much as you can.

An elective cesarean birth won't save you any time or energy. You might know the date of your child's birth ahead of time, but it *is* major abdominal surgery. It'll take you at least six to eight weeks afterwards to recover from it. And most of your recovery will be in your home—with your newborn baby. You'll need your partner, a postpartum doula, or a friend to help take care of you for the first few weeks. If you live in a home with stairs, you won't be able to use the stairs much for two weeks. You'll be learning the new skill of mothering and breastfeeding, *while you recover* from major abdominal surgery. Recovery after a vaginal birth ranges from one to two weeks.

But sometimes a cesarean birth is necessary. When it is necessary, it can be lifesaving for you and your baby. Before you agree to a cesarean birth, make sure that your caregiver has explained to you the medical indications that make it necessary. Also, make sure you understand and agree with him.

The Five Stays

One way to do your best to avoid a cesarean is to follow the "five stays:"

1. Stay healthy
2. Stay home as long as possible (during labor)
3. Stay upright (during labor)
4. Stay away from *unnecessary* interventions
5. Stay away from *uninformed* decision making

How will the five stays help you?

If you *stay healthy*—take the necessary dietary supplements, eat well, and exercise appropriately—you'll be in good shape for the birth and have fewer interventions. Some helpful exercises include doing Kegels, lunging or squatting (make sure you have someone there to spot you), walking, and swimming in moderation. Women who regularly do yoga may find that the flexibility and strength it gives them is a plus during labor. Be sure to consult your care provider about which exercises are right for you.

Staying home as long as possible during your labor means that you'll be further along in the active stage of labor before you leave your comfortable home environment and enter your birth place. At home you can move around without monitors. The sounds you hear will be the sounds of your own home. You can shower or bathe in your own tub. If you have pets at home, stroking your dog or cat can be very calming, and you can't do that once you've left. Also, the shorter the time you spend in the hospital before you give birth, the less likely you'll be treated as a *patient*. This will help you avoid unnecessary interventions that can slow or stop labor. If you go in later, you'll be treated like a *birthing mother*, which is what you are aiming for.

Staying upright during labor is very helpful. Upright positions use gravity to help the baby move down lower in your pelvis. The lower your baby is, the more your baby's head can change and open your cervix, preparing you for birth. Many moms tell us that while they were upright and could move freely, they felt more like a laboring mother and less like a patient. This freedom helped them postpone or do without an epidural.

Stay away from *unnecessary* interventions. For example, you might not need an epidural. If you can avoid an epidural or avoid pitocin inductions or augmentations, do so. They *are* helpful if they're needed. But consider whether the effects of the intervention are worth the possible side effects on you, your baby, and your labor. (See Chapter 6 for more on epidurals.)

Stay away from *uninformed* decision making. If you know what your choices truly are, then you can make the best decision possible. Being uninformed can lead to feelings of regret and negative birth memories that can last for years.

If you follow the *five stays*, you'll know you've done your best to avoid an unnecessary cesarean birth.

Techniques for Trying to Turn a Breech Baby

Just a few decades ago, doctors were used to delivering breech babies vaginally. Most doctors today are not trained in the technique. If your doctor or midwife is not well versed in breech vaginal birth, it could cause real dangers to your baby. Many doctors advise that a persistent breech baby have a cesarean birth. In order to avoid this, here are several methods different mothers have tried to turn a breech baby:

- Talk or play music and shine a flashlight at the vagina. The baby can hear the voice and see the light. Encourage the baby to go toward the light. It's easier if your partner does this, since you may not be able to reach.

- Use the knees-to-chest position (buttocks in the air). Do this next to a chair or on your bed. Be sure that you can easily get up from this position or have someone spot you. After being in this position for about 10 minutes, quickly kneel. The baby's head is the heaviest part and quickly getting up helps move the head down using gravity.

- Webster Technique: This is a chiropractic technique that does not touch the abdomen, but instead gently adjusts the spine. Make sure the chiropractor you see is used to working on pregnant women and is well versed in the Webster Technique. You may have to be adjusted several times for this to work.

- Moxibustion is an acupuncture technique using herbs. Find an acupuncturist who has experience in this technique. The technique encourages the baby to move, but it is not intended to get the baby to move if moving would not work (for example, if the cord is around the baby's neck or the cord is too short for the baby to change positions).

- Hypnosis is another way women can be encouraged to move their babies. Find a hypnotist or hypnobirthing instructor who is used to working with pregnant women. They can teach you self hypnosis to help move the baby.

External Version – The OB Method

If the above low tech methods do not turn your baby, ask your doctor about an *external version*. An OB will do this, usually in the hospital. They use an ultrasound to guide them and to be certain the cord isn't around the baby's neck. The doctor uses her hands on your stomach to move the baby into the head down (vertex) position. The ultrasound confirms when this is accomplished. This sounds like a serious thing to do, but think about it carefully before deciding. If your baby is still breech and a version turns him head down, you can have a vaginal birth and save yourself six to eight weeks of recovery from abdominal surgery. Make sure your doctor is experienced at external version. If your doctor is not comfortable with doing it, have her refer you to a doctor she knows who is experienced at it.

Remember, if you can avoid a cesarean birth, not only will your recovery from this birth be faster and easier, you will not have to worry about having a VBAC (Vaginal Birth after Cesarean) for your next birth. Many doctors and hospitals are not encouraging VBAC's and more women are having repeat cesarean births. If it is possible for you to have a safe vaginal birth—go for it!

When a Cesarean Birth Is Necessary—
It Can Still Be a Woman-Centered Birth

If medical circumstances require you to have a cesarean birth, you should still have a birth vision. Use your birth vision to make your birth as woman-centered as possible. You might need to schedule a cesarean birth ahead of time. That will give you the time to adjust to your circumstances and think about how to make your day special. Remember, you're not just going into surgery. You are becoming a mother and a family that day.

Pack a pillow or pillowcase from your house that smells like home. Have your partner or doula rub your feet and hands with lotion before you go into the operating room (OR). Bring a travel-sized ocean sound machine or music into the OR to help relax you.

Discuss the procedure with your doctor and ask any questions you may have to the anesthesiologist. Make sure that your partner and your doula can accompany you into the OR. Let them know you'd like birthing pictures, as well as pictures of your baby, right after he is born.

Talk to the nurse manager ahead of time about not being separated from your baby while you are in the recovery area. If there are no medical concerns about your baby, you will want him with you constantly. If you can hold him and nurse him within the first hour or so, you will start your recovery sooner. One of the biggest complaints we hear from mothers who have had a cesarean birth is that they were separated from their babies too long. Even two hours seems like forever when you have been waiting so long to see and hold your baby.

Take advantage of the *belly binder*—a wide Velcro girdle that gives your stomach muscles stability in the first few days after birth. It is very helpful when you get into or out of bed, or when you walk around. Ask your care provider to prescribe one for you. Remember to support your belly with your hands or a pillow and roll out of bed (don't sit straight up).

Take advantage of rooming-in with your baby. It will help you get a good start on nursing, and you'll feel less anxiety because you won't be separated from your baby. Make sure you have comfortable clothes and that you have your family and friends visit you, if that will be a comfort to you—or that they know to stay away, if you suspect you'll need your rest more. Cheerful flowers and chocolates are usually appreciated, too!

Phone the hospital's lactation consultants right away. Have as many appointments with them while you are in the hospital as you can. They can assist you if you need help and give you vital reassurance when nursing is going well. Every new mom has nursing questions.

When a Vaginal Birth Becomes a Cesarean Birth

Many women start having a vaginal birth that becomes a cesarean birth after long work and complications. It's helpful for any pregnant mother to have part of her birth vision discuss her desires in the event of a cesarean birth. Underline your wish for your doula and partner to both attend you. Also, underline your wish not to be separated from your baby unless his health necessitates it.

Our Clients' Suggestions for Recovering from a Cesarean:

If you feel you missed the moment after birth where they place your new baby on your chest, try this. Have your husband present your baby to you while lying in bed, sitting in the tub, or somewhere else you might have given birth if you had done it vaginally. A nude mother and baby can really help recapture those first missed moments of skin-to-skin. It can be healing and joyous. Be sure to nurse!

Wear silky pajamas—they help you slide out of bed more easily while recuperating.

Put a small refrigerator and microwave in your bedroom and stay on that floor for the first several days at home. Limiting steps is a good idea.

Use a mirror and look at your incision daily, so you can keep an eye on healing. Or, ask your partner. It's easier if you are lying down.

Limit visitors and length of visits, stay in your nightgown, yawn a lot, don't offer refreshments to visitors, leave the room to nurse or take a nap with your baby. They'll get the idea.

Having a Safe Vaginal Birth after Cesarean or VBAC

If your first birth was a cesarean birth, start thinking about your VBAC (Vaginal Birth after Cesarean) choices as soon as you can in your next pregnancy. Your birth team is crucial for a successful VBAC. A doula with VBAC experience is very important for encouragement and suggestions.

Choose your care provider very carefully. Make certain your doctor or midwife is willing to support you in having a VBAC. Here's what to look for in a care provider and birth facility:

- Find out what percentage of successful VBACs your facility has. Go to a hospital or birth center that has a good percentage of successful VBACs.

- Find out what kind of water you can use during your labor. Does the room have a shower or bath? A bath is very helpful in helping you to avoid an epidural. It is also helpful to have telemetric or doppler monitoring during your stay in the tub, so you won't have to get in and get out to be monitored. Having a heparin lock instead of an IV can also help. An IV limits mobility.

One of the keys to having a successful VBAC is avoiding an epidural if possible. It is crucial during a VBAC that you are able to push to the very best of your ability. You will also need to be able to move around and change positions during pushing. Having an epidural in place makes both of these more difficult. Instead, use the shower or tub.

Try to avoid a medical induction if you can. It's not nice to rush Mother Nature, especially when trying to accomplish a VBAC. If you and the baby remain healthy, going into labor naturally gives you the greatest chance of avoiding interventions which can lead to a repeat cesarean birth. Some practices won't use pitocin for a VBAC and some won't use cervidil or cervical ripeners, so check that out with your care provider, as well.

During a VBAC, it is important not to relive the problem that led to the last cesarean birth. This may take some mental preparation before the birth and extra support when that same point of dilation occurs. Doulas are a great help because they can support you through that emotional time.

Ask your doctor or midwife:

- How high-risk is my birth considered?
- How do you support a mom during a VBAC?
- Are you comfortable supporting *me* in a VBAC?
- When in pregnancy would you want to induce me?
- Can my labor be monitored with a doppler or waterproof telemetry while I'm in the tub?
- What medical indications would lead you to schedule a second cesarean?
- How many successful VBACs does your practice do yearly?
- Can I have a heparin lock instead of an IV?

Weighing the Risks and Benefits

Many women have had successful VBACs. Women often say they felt so much better after their VBAC than after their cesarean birth, even if they hadn't thought the cesarean birth was so bad. After all, the birth of your baby is generally a joyful event and cesareans can be joyful, too.

Benefits of a VBAC

Recovery time is so much shorter, and now you're mothering more than one child. The recovery time for a cesarean birth is around eight weeks. The recovery time for a vaginal birth is around two weeks. Having a vaginal birth makes it easier to have more children. Often one successful VBAC will lead to another. Cesarean births can limit the number of children you can safely have. Vaginal birth is usually far safer than surgical birth for both mother and baby.

Some Risks of VBAC

Doctors are concerned with uterine rupture along the original uterine suture site. The percentage is small, but the risk does exist. However, any woman in labor has some risk of uterine rupture, whether she trying to have a VBAC or not. There is also the risk of laboring long and then having another cesarean birth.

Do Your Emotional Work

Every woman who has had a cesarean birth has the fear that she'll need another cesarean. Work on overcoming your fears before labor. Have confidence in yourself. Hire a birth doula who will cheer you on in labor and help you to get past your previous stopping point.

Some women choose to plan a second cesarean for medical reasons. Perhaps the baby is breech and can't be turned, or the mother's health has become high-risk. There might be a cord or placenta problem. Or the baby's chest measurement is much larger than the head circumference, which could result in the shoulders getting stuck at birth.

The most important thing is to trust the dialogue you have with your care provider. If you're confident in your information and you choose a cesarean birth for good medical reasons, you can be confident that you are one of the small percentage of women who need a cesarean birth. Then you can be happy that your baby's health is protected and you are cared for. Pick a surgeon who is excellent at performing the surgery, and then make sure you have very good postpartum care when you're recovering at home.

Chapter 10

Breastfeeding is Bestfeeding

Cindy was trying to decide how to feed her baby, who was due to be born in about a month. She knew from the little she had read that breastmilk was better for the baby, but why even bother with nursing if she had to return to work in three months?

But at a friend's urging, she decided to research it more, so she could make an informed decision. After all, this was her baby, and his health was of prime importance to her. So, she looked on the internet, read a couple of more books, and attended a breastfeeding class.

Cindy also went to her nearby La Leche League gathering to meet the leader and see other women breastfeed. She got lots of tips on how she could make breastfeeding feasible while working. She discovered ways to have a career and still nurse for a year or even longer. The leader explained that Cindy's boss would appreciate how her breastfed baby would be healthier, which meant she would need to take fewer sick days off. While there, she also asked the other moms about baby doctors who were pro-breastfeeding, so she could concentrate on interviewing them. Cindy was really glad that she had a built-in support system now.

While reading, Cindy was surprised to learn how amazing her breasts really are. She found out that milk produced after a premature baby is born is different from milk produced for a full-term baby. It is like breasts have brains and know to make more calorie-rich milk for smaller babies. Cindy also discovered that the skin-to-skin contact during breastfeeding helps regulate the baby's temperature. She found a long list of all the good things breastmilk does for her baby—like reducing the incidence of diabetes, heart disease, allergies, asthma, and obesity. And breastmilk gives the baby perfect nutrition and protective immunities right from the first nursing. Plus, the research actually showed that not only are breastfed babies healthier, they are also smarter!

Cindy read that nursing reduces cancers and osteoporosis for the mother, and right after the birth, reduces bleeding. Lastly, she considered formula's inconvenience, cost, and questionable ingredients (like high levels of estrogen in soy formula). Measuring, mixing, warming the bottle, and making the baby wait—all that wasn't what she really wanted.

Cindy imagined holding her baby in her arms, nursing in the middle of the night, with no cares in the world, but to love and to nourish her baby. The vision felt right to her and seemed so obvious…her decision was made. Cindy thought to herself, "Why doesn't every woman breastfeed?"

Why Breastfeed?

Nursing is more than just food for the baby: it's a relationship as well. You might say it's a way to continue the closeness developed during the pregnancy. The baby is nestled in your loving arms, feeling safe and being perfectly nourished at the same time. Heaven on earth!

Your breasts produce the perfect food for your baby. Human milk is made for human babies, just as cow's milk is made for calves, cat's milk is made for kittens, and whale's milk is made for baby whales. Mammals produce the perfect nourishment for their own offspring, and humans are no different. No artificial formula is as good as the milk your baby gets from you.

Nursing also continues the body-to-body connection from pregnancy. The closeness helps you fall in love with your baby. The hormones released actually encourage cuddling and create a feeling of relaxed euphoria for both of you. The breastfeeding relationship helps your baby learn to trust you—and you to know your baby.

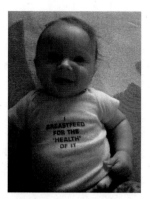

Jan's grandson, Zeev

Getting off to a Good Start

Most women worry about engorgement, nipple soreness, and adequate milk supply when, in fact, lack of education, confidence, and support are the greatest breastfeeding challenges.

The first thing you need to do before your baby is born is know where you're going to turn for breastfeeding help. Your doula can probably give you some help, and she can put you in touch with experts when you need them. You should also know how to get in touch with your local branch of La Leche League International (www.llli.org). If you'll have access to lactation consultants where you give birth, know who they are and how to reach them when you need them.

You need this support network in place before your baby is born because the single most important thing in breastfeeding success is your confidence that you can do it. It's easy to lose that confidence without strong support. So making sure that your support system is truly encouraging of breastfeeding is essential.

If your mother questions your choice to nurse or your partner doesn't want you to nurse in front of others, it will be harder to succeed. The best nutrition for your baby and a close connection to your baby far outweigh other people's discomfort or opinion. So make the special people in your life aware of the importance of successful breastfeeding to both you and your baby. And ask for their constant encouragement…especially if you waver. That can happen if you have very sore nipples or during the baby's first growth spurt, for example. Have your support people attend a breastfeeding class with you, so they can appreciate its value and learn as you do. That way, they can make suggestions or remind you that challenges are normal at first. People, patience, and perseverance will get you through early breastfeeding adjustments. It takes time to develop your particular style with your baby. This is why we often call it the "art of nursing."

You might be worried about breastfeeding because you've heard stories of mothers who tried to breastfeed and gave up. We won't try to tell you that you won't ever have problems, but we've found that the biggest problem women have with breastfeeding today is cultural.

Our culture just doesn't support breastfeeding. We live in a bottle-feeding culture. Just look around you: even in congratulations cards and gift wrap, a bottle is the symbol for baby. Even if your friends know you are going to breastfeed, you will probably receive bottles as gifts. Bottles and formula are everywhere. Formula companies spend big money to make it so. On the other hand, breastmilk is free, which doesn't make much of a corporate profit. How will this affect you, the breastfeeding new mother? You may be given free formula—just in case. Please, refuse it!

As a new breastfeeding mom, you may feel shy about breastfeeding in public. This is normal at first. But keep in mind, if some other young woman sees you discreetly nursing your baby in public with confidence, you may just influence her to breastfeed her baby when she has one. Try nursing in front of a mirror to see how much others can see of you and to perfect your technique. Your courage can help change our formula culture to a breastfeeding culture. Thank you!

Breastfeeding Books to Read Before the Birth

Here are some good books to help you breastfeed with confidence:
- *The Womanly Art of Breastfeeding* by La Leche League International. This book gives you good information about the ins and outs of breastfeeding. Remember, it is both an art and a science!

- *The Ultimate Breastfeeding Book of Answers: The Most Comprehensive Problem-Solving Guide to Breastfeeding from the Foremost Expert in North America* by Dr. Jack Newman and Teresa Pitman. This book helps you diagnose your problems and come up with good solutions.

- *The Breastfeeding Book: Everything You Need to Know about Nursing Your Child from Birth through Weaning* by Martha Sears and Dr. William Sears. They are excellent at helping you build attachment parenting and nursing skills.

The Three A's of Breastfeeding

The basics of successful breastfeeding aren't very complicated. We like to summarize them with three A's:

ALIGNMENT – Regardless of which position you hold your baby in, the baby's ear, shoulder and hip should be in a straight line to ensure proper swallowing. Positions to consider are: clutch (football) (Figure 48), cross-cradle (Figure 49), cradle, side-lying (Figure 50), Australian (Figure 51), and sitting. (Sitting is for later when your child can sit on your lap.) We often say to place the baby tummy-to-tummy (baby's against yours), with its buttocks tucked in close (to your body) and the baby at an angle (head at breast and feet on lap) for good positioning. Feeding at an angle, burping at an angle and placing baby at an angle after nursing can reduce reflux.

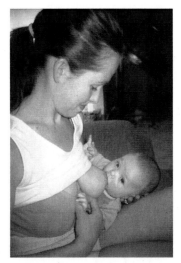

Figure 48. Clutch hold

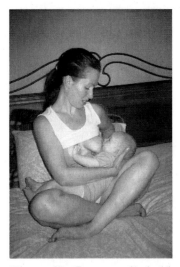

Figure 49. Cross-cradle hold

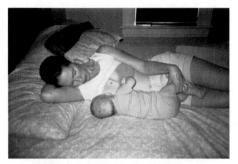

Figure 50. Sidelying nursing

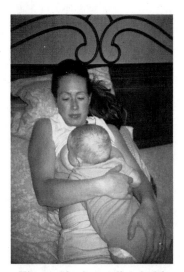

Figure 51. Australian hold

AREOLA – Get a good latch. More than just the nipple should be in the baby's mouth to prevent nipple soreness. *Good latch-on is critical.* Tickle the baby's lips with your nipple (while holding your breast with your hand in a c-shape). When baby's mouth is wide open (like a baby bird), bring baby onto the "bull's eye" and relax. Your areola darkens during pregnancy, so the baby can see it easily after birth. Avoid putting your breast into the baby's mouth, since this can lead to you having neck, shoulder, and back pain. Recliners, gliders with an ottoman, or a chair with a stool encourage you to lean back while nursing.

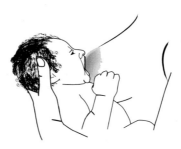

Figure 52. Asymmetric latch

Bring the baby onto the nipple from underneath the areola, making sure lips are flanged outward (like a fish's mouth). The baby's chin should be touching the breast and the nose should be just slightly away from the breast (Figure 52). Compression combined with suction is the goal, so you should feel a pulling or tugging sensation, not pain or pinching. If it's painful, break suction and start again. Pull down on the baby's chin when attaching (or afterwards) to help widen the mouth to ensure better latch-on. Do this using your index finger on the hand supporting the breast.

ACTIVE SUCK (colostrum) to **AUDIBLE SWALLOW** (breast milk): To feel confident that your baby is getting enough, look for rhythmic movement around the ear and jaw until the milk comes in (3 to 5 days after birth). Then listen for obvious sucking, gulping, and swallowing. New moms often worry about the baby getting enough in those first few days. The colostrum is thick and rich in fat and calories, so your baby doesn't need much to thrive. Have confidence in your breasts to do their job!

You and the baby will establish a nursing rhythm. The baby uses a suck, sigh (or pause), swallow pattern to feed. So don't expect constant breastfeeding—there will be pauses in the action. Plus, some babies are barracudas and others are grazers. Barracudas are vigorous nursers and strip the milk from the breast pretty efficiently. Grazers take their time and can be at the breast for a while until feeling satisfied. Your baby might be anywhere in between. Don't worry—you and your baby will figure it out!

How Not to Worry

It's common to have some difficulties when you're just starting to breastfeed. Millions of other women have faced the same challenges and overcome them. Here are a few problems you might be worried about, and some helpful ideas for solving them.

My Breasts Are Too Full

The breast, areola, and nipple are in transition after the birth. So engorgement and tender nipples don't necessarily mean you're doing something wrong. The breasts vigorously filling with milk can be uncomfortable, but you should be proud that your body is doing its job. You have the perfect way to decrease the fullness—your baby! If your breasts are too full to latch the baby on, try these ideas:

- Warm shower or warm compresses on breasts
- Breast massage (like during self-exam)
- Hand expression to relieve some fullness
- Pumping to relieve some fullness

During nursing, you can gently stroke your breast or do compressions, encouraging the milk toward the nipple. And, in between feedings, use cold compresses to help with uncomfortable swelling if you have it. Frozen peas in a bag work really well! Using washed, raw cabbage leaves in your bra for a short period is a tried and true way of reducing engorgement. Talk to a professional about it, however, because it can lead to production problems if used incorrectly.

My Nipples Are Sore

Some women have sore nipples, some don't. Some did with their first, but not their second. Every nursing experience is different. Sore nipples are common, but they are not normal! Breastfeeding should not hurt. Keep these basics in mind to help avoid, diminish, or treat sore nipples:

- Make sure you have a deep latch.
- Break suction of the latch with your little finger—to protect the nipple tissue.
- Air dry—so nipple is not moist.
- Avoid drying substances on breast (such as soap or alcohol), which could lead to cracking and bleeding.
- Start on least sore side—baby is most hungry at first.
- Rub a couple of drops of breast milk gently onto the nipple after feeding—it has natural healing properties.
- Use a pure lanolin product nipple cream—it helps with healing.
- Wear a breast shell in your bra occasionally—to protect and heal nipples.

Remember, latch, latch, latch! Your baby's latch should be correct each time you nurse. Most sore nipples happen because you're not using a good latch. Have your doula, La Leche League leader, or lactation consultant watch you nurse and help you perfect your latch. Nursing is not supposed to hurt. Once you're confident in latching on your baby, sore nipples should be a thing of the past. If they are not, please see a lactation consultant for an evaluation because there is another reason for your sore nipples.

Do I Have Enough Milk?

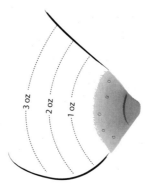

Figure 53. If only breasts had ounce markers...

This is the age-old question all new mothers ask. The short answer is yes, you do. If women had clear breasts with little red ounce markers, we'd all breastfeed with confidence (Figure 53). You'd see how much the baby is getting. Remember that the size of your breasts doesn't determine the milk supply: the baby's demand for it does.

We're asking you to have faith in your ability to supply milk for the baby's demands. But we're also asking you to drink a lot of fluids, eat well, and sleep enough, so you can breastfeed successfully and mother adequately. Milk doesn't need to be one of those fluids. You don't need to drink milk to make milk. Have you ever seen a mother cow drinking milk?

Is My Baby Getting Enough?

Your baby may have only one or two wet diapers during the first day or two after birth.

Beginning about the third or fourth day, your baby will have at least five to six wet diapers (if you're using disposable diapers).

He will pass meconium, the greenish-black, tarry first stool, over the first day or two. Your baby will begin having at least two to five bowel movements a day beginning about the third day after birth.

Ask yourself: Is he active and vigorous when awake? Is he dehydrated? Gently pinch the skin on the back of baby's hand: does it go back quickly? Is the soft spot on his head sunken (sunken may mean dehydrated)? Is his mouth wet or dry? Is his urine yellow (brick-dust color indicates dehydration)?

If you suspect your baby is dehydrated, call his doctor right away. Most babies will get enough milk if their latch-on is correct.

Let Your Baby Be Your Guide

The baby will be your best guide in letting you know when and how long to nurse. But to give you a rough idea, you might want to let the baby nurse for about 20 minutes on one side each feeding.

Think of it this way—it takes about 15 to 20 minutes to eat dinner, right? So consider the first breast you offer the baby to be dinner. After active feeding for 20 minutes or so on one side, the baby has gotten plenty of fat and calories. Active feeding means feeling deep tugging in your breast and seeing the suck, sigh, swallow pattern. Burp and change the baby, and then offer dessert—the other breast. Sometimes we want one piece of apple pie, sometimes we want two helpings, and sometimes we pass on dessert completely.

If your baby nurses well on one side for 20 minutes, that's fine. Recent research suggests that babies gain better if they spend 20 minutes on one side at a feeding, rather than 10 minutes on each side. Just offer the fuller one at the next feeding. If your baby nurses for 20 minutes or more on both sides, that is fine, too. Breastfed babies don't overeat, so let them guide you as to how long to nurse.

Please don't spend too much time watching the clock. It's more important that he's nursing vigorously and latching well than how many minutes it takes.

If the baby is not nursing vigorously or takes a lot of breaks, try using breast compressions. This will encourage milk to flow into his mouth for active sucking and swallowing. To do breast compressions, hold your breast with your hand in a C shape, well above the areola. Squeeze and hold your breast. Keep the gentle pressure on until your baby stops sucking, even with the compression, and then repeat. This is different from hand expression or massaging your breast.

Am I Feeding Often Enough?

Some care providers will want you to be a clock watcher. Others will say to follow the baby's cues. What cues? Well, rooting for the nipple, opening wide, sucking on fingers, and crying are all pretty good signs.

Most breastfeeding experts recommend nursing a newborn on-cue, at least 8 to 10 times a day for the first two weeks. This generally results in good weight gain. If you allow the baby to sleep longer between feedings at night, be sure to make up for that during the day by offering the breast more often. These frequent feedings will contribute to fatigue during your postpartum period, no doubt. But remember, all new babies are up often to eat no matter how they are fed!

Practice nursing while lying down. Once you hone that skill, night-time nursing will disturb your sleep much less. Try lying down for a nap during the day and nursing your baby. It takes several tries to figure out whether you need a pillow under your baby or a pillow under your breast. You can use the breast closest to the bed or the higher breast. Keep practicing until you and your baby are good at it. Then night nursing will be a breeze!

The baby's tummy is only the size of its fist, so not much will fit in. And breastmilk is so easily digested that babies are hungry again quite soon. The digestibility of breastmilk results in a laxative effect on the baby's first bowel movement (meconium). This helps the baby rid his body of bilirubin, which is carried out through the stool to help avoid newborn jaundice. The stool will go from a tarry, blackish looking substance to a transitional greenish stool, and then to the liquidy, mustard-yellow stool associated with nursing. There will probably be some seedy-looking things in the baby's diapers. They are undigested milk curds. It means you're giving the baby plenty of nutrition and what wasn't needed just passed through.

Ten Gentle Reminders

By now you should be confident that nursing is simple, natural, and easy. Here are a few hints to make it even easier.

1. Try to wash your hands before nursing. Use soap and water for the length of time it takes to sing Happy Birthday or the ABC song to ensure clean hands. You don't have to wash your breasts, however. The Montgomery glands do that cleansing for you. Aren't our bodies wonderful?

2. Use the skin-to-skin method whenever you can with the baby. Even if later, someone gives the baby a bottle of breastmilk, encourage skin-to-skin contact. Remember, try to avoid giving your baby bottles for the first three-to-four weeks to avoid nipple confusion. A great way to interact with the baby using skin-to-skin is during a bath or shower...take one together. Men, watch out, though, because the baby will grab your chest hairs!

3. Set up nursing stations on each level of the house. Consider having a comfortable place with lots of pillows for support (even if you have a nursing pillow) and a stool for your feet. Also have a drink or snack, facial tissue, burp cloth, blanket, a phone, and the TV remote handy.

4. Keeping the baby awake during frequent feedings can be a feat in itself in the first few days. Some hints: try baby exercises before nursing, like sit-ups and leg bicycles, unwrap baby so he's not too warm, gently scratch the top of his head to stimulate him, rub under his chin to encourage lapping of the milk, or pump the baby's arm. Sometimes changing his diaper will get his attention, too.

5. Weight gain pressures can be very anxiety producing. Many pediatricians want the baby to gain back their birth weight by two weeks old. (Babies often lose up to 10% of their birth weight right after the birth.) On the other hand, remember that many babies in America are formula-fed, and since formula is not as easily digestible as breastmilk, formula-fed babies usually gain weight more rapidly. Some breastfeeding experts make a persuasive argument that, instead of worrying whether breastfed babies are gaining weight as fast as formula-fed babies, doctors should be asking whether the formula-fed babies' rapid weight gain is such a good thing.

Consider These Weight-Gain Questions:

- Could there have been human error in reading or recording your baby's birth weight?

- How many different scales has your baby been weighed on?

- Were these scales properly and recently calibrated?

- Was your baby always weighed without a diaper?

- Why should you worry about weight loss before your milk comes in?

- Won't the baby gain more during the first growth spurt?

- What guide is your baby's doctor using for weight gain and loss? Was it based on formula-fed babies?

- Did anyone consider individual growth patterns, due to genetic makeup and personal uniqueness?

6. Growth spurts will occur at around 7–10 days, 3 weeks, 6 weeks, 3 months, and 6 months. This is when the baby puts a greater demand on your supply to meet its growing needs. Growth spurts usually last two days and require a lot from the mother. So spend those two days in bed with the baby sleeping, eating, drinking, and falling in love some more. We call this "babymooning" (like honeymooning, but with your baby).

7. Try not to use a pacifier, bottle, or pump until your milk supply is well established and you're feeling more confident. In the beginning, you can hand-express some milk. Pumping can really contribute to sore nipples and uses up a lot of valuable time. Use a clean finger as a natural pacifier for babies who seem to have a strong sucking urge. Pacifiers or bottles can contribute to nipple confusion, so consider avoiding both until after the 3-week growth spurt. Even the American Academy of Pediatrics (AAP) recommends waiting until after the 3-week growth spurt to introduce a pacifier to reduce the incidence of SIDS. A baby can be given breastmilk by dropper, syringe, spoon, or cup.

8. If you use a bottle for breastmilk, have someone else feed the baby initially. The baby will smell you close by and prefer you to the bottle. Smart baby! Also, warm the milk to body temperature by holding the bottle under warm running water, place in a pot of warm water, or use a bottle warmer. Never use the microwave, which heats unevenly and could leave dangerous hot spots in the milk. Use a nipple that encourages the baby to open wide and flange its lips, like with breastfeeding. And last, change sides after giving half the bottle (and burping and changing). This allows for more equal eye-hand coordination to develop in the baby. Plus, don't forget the skin-to-skin factor discussed above. Why not copy some of the benefits associated with breastfeeding when using a bottle? Share these hints with any of the baby's caretakers and be sure to remind them to never prop a bottle during feedings. Never leave a bottle unattended with the baby because the baby could choke.

9. Sometimes you might have an untimely letdown of your milk. Maybe you're grocery shopping and you hear a baby cry three aisles away. All of a sudden, you feel a tingly sensation in your breasts and the milk starts to flow. If you wore nursing pads in your bra, good. If not, putting gentle pressure on your nipples (pressing with the inside of your wrists or crossing your arms and pressing) will cause the milk to stop. Helpful hint: if a pad is sticking to your nipple, put a few drops of warm water on that spot and gently peel the pad off. Consider not using the adhesive strip on disposable pads, since the pad will be attached to the bra. If it's also stuck to you, the nipple will be damaged when pulling the bra flap down. Some women find washable cotton pads the most comfortable.

10. Sexuality is a little bit affected by nursing. Breastfeeding women have dryer vaginas because of hormonal factors. So keep a water-soluble lubricant in your bedside table for intercourse. It can be purchased in the feminine hygiene aisle at your local pharmacy. Be sure to discuss all family planning options with your healthcare provider.

Lactational Amenorrhea Method

According to the Lactational Amenorrhea Method, if a mother can answer "no" to the following questions, then there is only a 1-2% chance of pregnancy:

1. Has your period returned?

2. Are you supplementing regularly or allowing long periods without nursing either day or night?

3. Is your baby more than six months old?

Summing It All Up

As in the rest of this book, we're encouraging you to have confidence in your body. Breasts have nourished all kinds of mammals for hundreds of thousands of years. Watch your baby's cues and listen to her messages. Keep the basics in mind to achieve successful breastfeeding. And remember, you are the one to determine your own success. Any breastmilk that you provide for your baby is the best gift you can give her. Not only does the breastfeeding connection ensure a healthier baby, it contributes to the ever-important trust relationship between mother and child.

Chapter 11

Preparing for Your New Life at Home

Barb arrived home from the hospital with her hubby and their new daughter. Her mom and dad hadn't gotten in from out of town yet, so the house was quiet and empty. They were going to stay for the weekend to meet the new baby.

It was 2:00 PM and Barb's stomach was growling. The baby wouldn't stop crying and daddy was busy unloading the car. She could smell a messy diaper, but couldn't seem to find any changing stuff. She took the baby upstairs and discovered that the baby's supplies were still in bags in the closet and her newborn clothes weren't in the drawer. She had asked her husband to set up the basics in the nursery and to do one load of wash.

When he joined her upstairs, she asked about diapers and onesies. He thought she meant set up the crib, not set up supplies, and he did the wash, but it hadn't been dried yet.

It was time to nurse, so she took the baby downstairs to find the diaper bag and the nursing pillow. The diaper bag had been left in the car, so Barb sat on the sofa breastfeeding her unchanged baby, holding back the tears while her husband went back outside. The clothes were still wet.

All right, it's your turn. Get out a marker and highlight everything that's wrong with this story!

Here are some of the things we noticed:

1.   No one was there to help upon arrival at home.

2.   Company was coming to meet the baby, not to help.

3.   The mother was hungry.

4.   The dad was not attending to the mom's needs, even though he was helping.

5.   Baby supplies had not been arranged before the birth.

6. The mother had to go upstairs.

7. The nursery had not been set up.

8. The baby's clothes had not been washed or put away.

9. There was miscommunication.

10. Nursing stations had not been set up.

11. The mom was feeling overwhelmed.

12. And the clothes were still wet!

So you might want to think about these issues:

1. Decide what kind of help you want at home and how soon you will need it.

2. Avoid having *company* in the first two weeks; instead, have them visit to help *you*.

3. Make casseroles to freeze ahead and arrange for friends to bring meals.

4. Discuss your priorities and plan for baby and mother-care beforehand.

5. Buy newborn supplies and arrange them for your convenience a month before your due date (in case the baby is born early). Concentrate on your baby's immediate needs, like clothes, diapers, and a cozy place to sleep (a co-sleeper or bassinet). There will be plenty of time to handle the rest of it later.

6. Limit your activities in early postpartum; rest and recover.

7. Think about what items you will really need *from the beginning*. The baby will probably not be sleeping in the nursery at the start. A well supplied changing station on each level of your house is what you need.

8. Organize your baby's first clothes and have them ready for his homecoming. If you didn't get that done, you could ask a friend or family member to do it for you during your hospital stay.

9. Communicate your wishes calmly and thoroughly. Don't assume your support system will know how you want things done. Many new moms keep a list on the refrigerator of things they need help with that day. When someone visiting offers to help, ask them to choose something from the refrigerator list.

10. Arrange a comfortable place to nurse your baby on every level of your house.

11. Know that sometimes, feeling overwhelmed comes with the territory. Take care of yourself first. Remember that you will need to eat and rest, so that you can mother well.

12. Wash, wash, wash! Babies go through lots of clothes.

A Well-Stocked Changing Station:

- Waterproof pads
- Disposable changing sheets
- Newborn diapers
- Wipes or wash cloth, soap and water
- Diaper rash ointment
- Alcohol & cotton swab or cotton balls (for cord care)
- Petroleum jelly and gauze pads (for circumcision)
- Baby lotion for massages
- Change of clothes
- Burp cloths
- Blankets

Help! I Need Somebody
(as the Beatles Would Say)

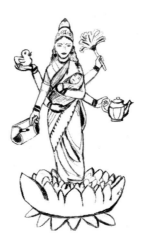

Figure 54. When you need a hand, the postpartum doula is there

Getting help before, during, and after the baby came is what women did for generations. Family help may be less available in these modern times, so consider professional help if necessary (Figure 54). As we've discussed in this book already, help comes in many forms, so appropriate assistance is out there for everybody.

Letting others help you is another issue. Many women are fiercely independent these days. They're used to doing it all. Why not allow people to help when you really need it? It's a good life lesson. It teaches you about recognizing limits, trusting in others, and the value of mutual generosity. You really don't need to be wonder woman!

Many people casually mention bringing you a casserole for when the baby comes home, but we often think it's an empty offer. Think differently. Why not help others to help you by giving them direction? Here's how.

Baby Shower Advice

During your baby shower, have your **Postpartum Help** sheet out (we've included one at the end of this chapter) for those who are truly interested in helping you transition into being a new family. Have the greeter tell the guests about the sheet and ask them to fill it in while making name tags. Be sure to have a few names and offers on the list before most guests arrive to give them an idea of what they could offer.

Those attending the baby shower often say, "I wish someone had done this for me when I was a new mother!" It just feels right to help other women through this rite of passage into motherhood—that's why we're doulas!

This can also be done for women who are not having showers. A list is circulated through a neighborhood group, La Leche League group, mom's group, or church group—and *voilà!* The mother gets help.

A great idea to consider when making a gift list for your baby shower is to request a postpartum doula to be paid for by a group of friends. And if you are a repeat mom, friends and family are often looking for a gift that you don't already have. It's a gift that will never be returned!

Open Up

Communicating your wants and needs with your partner, immediate family, and close friends is essential. We often assume loved ones automatically know what we like, how we feel, or what we're thinking. You know what they say about assuming! Telling your partner what you expect help-wise and informing your family and friends of your specific needs before the baby comes is just being proactive. That *is* a good thing! You can always change your mind or adapt the situation later if need be. But just muddling your way through postpartum is not advisable.

Direct communication with visitors and well-wishers is also important. Be clear about how soon you want phone calls. As soon as the baby is born, people will want to visit, and you will want to show your beautiful baby to them. But be careful. You'll get tired more easily than you expect to. Also, your newborn can become easily over-stimulated by too many visitors who stay too long. Limit visits and visitors for the first two weeks to protect your baby and you. Wear a bathrobe during visits and yawn a lot. You probably won't have to fake being tired. Some women leave to nurse and just never come back—good hint!

Do *not* be a hostess in the early days. Be sure not to offer refreshments or your guests will stay too long. If they bring you some food, thank them, and tell them your family will enjoy it later that day. By limiting distractions, you recover faster, which means you can mother better—which is what everyone wants anyway.

Mommy Care

Don't forget about your needs as a new mother. Put together a personal care kit. You might want to include clean all-cotton underwear, a variety of pads and panty-liners, personal wipes, bidet bottle, analgesic cream (for stitches), hemorrhoid treatments, stool softener, sitz bath—if you brought it home from the hospital.

You will be given cold packs to use immediately after the birth. Some women need to use them when they get home if they still have swelling and pain. Many care providers recommend using warm and cold intermittently. Cold is for pain and swelling, while warmth promotes healing. Some midwives recommend taking maxi-pads, wetting them and applying comfrey, then freezing them in the shape of a bowl. Check with your healthcare provider about using herbs.

Red Means Stop

The vaginal bleeding after birth is called *lochia*. At first, it's heavier than a period, and you may see some clots. By the time you leave the hospital, it's similar to having a period. As the days go by, you should notice less lochia, the color should change to pink, and then to brown. Brown indicates healing at the placental site. To avoid uterine infection (and pregnancy), avoid unprotected intercourse until the lochia is brown. Many doctors and midwives recommend avoiding tampons or tub baths until the lochia turns brown. If the lochia reverts back to red, or suddenly increases in amount, your body is telling you that you are doing too much. Make sure to take it very easy the next day.

Breastfeeding Doesn't Require Much Equipment

You've got the right equipment—your breasts! So, let's talk about products that support the equipment: bras and pads. Here are the basics to consider:

When to buy? – Most educators and consultants recommend getting the bra toward the end of the pregnancy or right after birth. This way, it's newer and will be a good fit. Nursing bras are made to expand a bit to accommodate the changing breast, so you don't need to worry about that.

How many? – We suggest at least three bras.

What size? – Measure around the back, under the arms, and above the breasts (across the breastbone) to determine band size. Then measure around the back and across the widest part of your bust. The difference between these two numbers determines your cup size. One inch – A cup, 2 inches – B cup, 3 inches – D cup, 4 inches – DD cup, and so on. Having a lactation counselor or consultant fit you is a great help.

What style? – Avoid underwire bras that can put pressure on milk glands or ducts, which could cause a problem. Choose a fabric that's right for you and be sure the straps are sturdy. Stretchy ones can lose support ability. How the flaps open and close are very important. You want to feel efficient at doing that maneuver!

What care is needed? – Since you'll be washing your bras often, wash them by hand in a mild detergent. Air-dry them to maintain the best elasticity and support. There are lots of choices now, so nursing bras can be functional, fun, and feminine.

What about pads? – If you find you are leaking, your first choice is what type of pad to use–disposable or washable. If you use disposable ones, be sure there is no plastic to trap moisture and don't use the adhesive strip. Milk can dry and cause the pad to stick to the nipple. If you pull the bra flap down and the pad is stuck to the cup, the pad will pull nipple skin off and contribute to nipple soreness. If the pad sticks, dribble warm water on the pad and carefully peel it off your nipple. Any cotton material can be used, like cut-up hankies or diapers, but there are washable nursing pads on the market as well. They can be thrown in the washer with the baby's clothes. Regardless of type, change your pads frequently.

To Pump or Not to Pump

Pump questions are always asked in breastfeeding classes. It's probably best not to get a pump until after you've had the baby and are actually nursing.

Hand expression has become less popular, but it worked for hundreds of thousands of years. It's an easy combination of positioning your hand on the breast, pressing towards the chest wall and then rolling your thumb towards the nipple. These motions copy the baby's nursing mechanics without making your nipples sore. So try it—you'll like it!

When the three-week growth spurt is over, decide what your true needs are and then make your purchase. Pumps can cost up to $400, so consider your selection carefully because they are non-returnable. And you should not use someone else's pump for health and hygiene reasons.

Many women get the hand-held pump often covered by insurance before leaving the hospital. Not a bad idea. However, there are also electric and hospital-grade pumps. So gather the facts and talk to professionals who offer pumps for sale or rent to determine what fits your lifestyle best. How you plan on using the pump (how often, where, etc.) and what's available in your community are the two main factors to explore.

Other Tools

Sometimes a lactation consultant or counselor is needed to advise you on other tools that may help you succeed with breastfeeding. A supplemental nursing system may be used to help a baby gain weight or nipple shields might be suggested for pre-term babies, for instance. If you are thinking about giving up breastfeeding because of unusual or difficult circumstances, get the help you need to persevere. Using devices that will ensure the best nutrition for your baby will be well worth the effort you made.

Who's Who in Breastfeeding Help

There are people formally educated in helping with breastfeeding. A family doctor or pediatrician might also be an IBCLC (Internationally Board Certified Lactation Consultant). This is an important credential for a doctor, nurse, or lactation consultant to have. Try to find a doctor for your baby who is an IBCLC or who has one on their staff.

Others who may be of help are Certified Lactation Counselors (CLC). They too have completed all requirements to maintain a certified status to provide nursing assistance.

There are also La Leche League leaders ready to help you. They are volunteers who have breastfeed their own babies successfully and then gone through La Leche League's program to become a volunteer helper. And don't forget about your doula!

Others with experience and enthusiasm can help, too. If your mom breastfed you or you have friends who breastfed, they can be a great source of support. Try to find good, constructive breastfeeding support before you give birth.

What to Look for in a Doctor

The doctor or midwife you are seeing for prenatal care is probably not the one who will be seeing you or your baby after the birth. How do you choose a doctor?

First: Decide what *kind* of doctor you want. A family physician is one choice which has the advantage of the doctor knowing your whole family, inside and out. You'll also have the added advantage of being able to question the doctor about you or other family members while the baby is having a check-up.

Or choose a pediatrician. A pediatrician will see just your baby, but is a baby specialist. Be sure you are clear on their care philosophy and practices. Asking for a guide booklet they often provide is a good idea. That way, the baby really does come with a manual.

Second: Ask your friends with babies whom they recommend and why. Try to find a doctor who is also a lactation consultant, since breastfeeding questions are usually the most common for an otherwise healthy baby.

Third: Interview two or three doctors at least two months before your baby is due.

Some possible questions:

1. Are you a lactation consultant, or do you have one on staff?

2. How many children do you have and how many were breastfed?

3. What is your practice regarding immunizations? (You should be able to have a dialogue with your doctor about immunizations, addressing your concerns, and coming up with a mutually supported solution.)

4. Can I bring my baby for a "nurse" or "well-baby" visit? (These are good for weigh-ins, if necessary, and also for immunizations without making a doctor's appointment.)

5. How do you feel about baby weight gain, especially in breastfed babies? (A doctor should look at many factors of your baby's health, only one of which is weight gain.)

6. How does your office handle after-hours calls?

Last: The most important thing is for you to feel comfortable discussing issues with your doctor. Any doctor who intimidates you or does not allow you time to ask questions and get them answered is not the doctor for you.

Can I Still Breastfeed if I Need Prescription Drugs?

If you need to take a prescription drug while breastfeeding, check with your local La Leche League chapter. They have good breastfeeding-and-drug reference books. Many drugs can be safely taken while breastfeeding. Work with your doctor and let him know how important breastfeeding is to you. You rarely need to pause or stop breastfeeding to take the drugs you need safely. A great resource is *Medications and Mothers' Milk* by Thomas W. Hale, PhD.

If you need to take an antidepressant for postpartum depression, for example, there are some drugs you can use while breastfeeding. Don't make the mistake of suffering with postpartum depression and not getting help because you are breastfeeding. If you do develop depression, get help! A mother can nurse and still take antidepressants. It is very important for you to be able to mother your baby to the very best of your ability. See your doctor and get help. Your baby will thank you!

Remember that some simple over-the-counter drugs may be inappropriate while breastfeeding. For example, decongestants might reduce your milk supply. If you have a question about an over-the-counter medicine, ask your La Leche League leader, lactation consultant, or pharmacist.

A Little Bit on Postpartum Depression

The majority of women will experience the baby blues. It's caused by fatigue, family adjustments, and new responsibilities. Sometimes it's genetic. If you or someone in your family has a history of depression, you're more likely to experience it. So, with the baby blues, you may cry a little bit, doubt your ability to mother well, and miss the pre-baby life you had.

Postpartum depression is more serious: it affects the woman's whole lifestyle. For example, crying would be more frequent and intense. Behavior and reactions are out of the ordinary. A depressed woman can experience physical changes or pain. These things and others can make her feel very out of control and like less of a mother. She needs help.

Postpartum psychosis is the extreme case of depression. It involves a break with reality. Immediate care is required to head off a crisis for the mother, baby, and family. Keep in mind that this serious condition is extremely rare.

At the end of this chapter is a chart that compares baby blues, postpartum depression, and postpartum psychosis. You'll also find a few questions to ask yourself that might help you see whether you're at risk. A week after birth, answer these. If there are signs of depression, get help! Don't feel embarrassed or ashamed. Postpartum depression can be serious. Your care provider should have numbers for support groups, therapists, and psychiatrists to refer you to if you need them. Treatments can range from a hot meal and a good night's sleep (for the baby blues) to hospitalization and specific treatments (for the rare cases of psychosis).

A postpartum doula is the ideal solution to help reduce the chances of experiencing depression. She can help make sure you consider these ten things:

1. Take good care of yourself—eat well (and regularly), drink lots of fluids, get enough sleep and have your needs attended to first.

2. Be flexible and not too hard on yourself.

3. Organize and prioritize to stay focused.

4. Get help, and remember to thank people who help you—especially new dads.

5. Go out and talk with other new moms—with or without your baby.

6. Treat yourself to something special—with or without your partner.

7. Try relaxation methods, meditation, or journaling.

8. Be with your baby for times of need *and* times of fun—like massage.

9. Increase activities slowly, and exercise when appropriate with doctor's approval.

10. Limit distractions during this time of adjustment to avoid overexertion—like too many visitors.

Help On Your Fridge!

Before you give birth, put these phone numbers on your fridge *and* in your birth bag:

- Your birth or postpartum doula's number.
- Your local La Leche League leader's number.
- Your local hospital's or your doctor's lactation consultant's number.
- The number of a local nursing warmline (get it from La Leche League).
- The number of a trusted friend who has breastfed successfully recently.
- The number of a local parenting warmline (get from hospital or La Leche League).

These helpful numbers will provide a line of support in case you need it. If you have a breastfeeding or parenting concern you usually need help right away. So call for help! A handy chart with spaces for all these numbers can be found at the end of the chapter.

The Best Way to Raise Your Child Is...

A great way to handle any advice is to say, "Thanks for your advice; we'll take it into consideration." If you like it, enter it into your parental data bank. If you don't, ignore it. Either way, the advice giver is answered and you are not committed to anything.

There are plenty of books out there telling you how to parent. Here are some of our personal reflections regarding parenthood:

- When you have a situation you don't know how to handle, pretend you are alone in a log cabin in the middle of nowhere with no way out or in and no way to communicate with the outside world because of a blizzard. This helps you remember to use your own ingenuity. You will figure out a solution that feels right for you.

- If you make an honest mistake with your newborn, try not to worry – he won't remember. And you won't be the first parent to do it.

- Always go with your gut – intuition exists! If it doesn't feel right, it isn't.

- Babies have these special antennae behind the soft spot on the top of their heads. They come up and sense whenever a mom is going to have *a hot meal, hot bath, or hot sex* – then the baby cries.

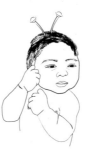

Hot meal, hot bath, or hot sex?

- If you have just fed, burped, changed, and checked on your baby's safety and loved your baby and he's still fussing, don't feel guilty about having that hot meal, bath, or sex. You should not lose yourself when you become a mom.

- Many problems occur around 2:00 AM when you are tired and cranky. Make a pledge with your partner not to make any serious decisions in the middle of the night. Use the light of day and make decisions when you are calmer.

- Try to get eight hours or more sleep within a twenty-four hour period. Your newborn will wake during the night, so you need to nap during the day, too.

- Each day with a newborn can seem incredibly long. But the weeks fly by quickly.

- Babies really do grow up before you know it, so cherish every minute you have with them. It's an amazing journey!

Adventures in Parenting

Try to prepare as well as you can in advance of the birth. That way, you can just keep falling in love with your baby as you recover. The story at the beginning of this chapter covers a variety of issues for you to consider. But always have a back-up plan. No matter how well you prepare, you can't control the universe! Something is bound to become a challenge, but that's life. Control what you can—just like during birth. But be open to change. Don't set your standards too high, since this is a time of change, recovery, and adjustment. That's a lot in itself. Parenthood is an adventure that lasts a lifetime, so take your time easing into it. You'll be fine!

Postpartum Emergency Information Sheet

Name: _____

Address: _____

Phone Numbers _____

Midwife/Obstetrician # _____

Pediatrician # _____

Family Practitioner # _____

Closest family or friend # _____

Emergency #s–

Police _____

Fire Department _____

Poison Control _____

Ambulance _____

Additional Names and Numbers

_____

_____

_____

_____

Special Instructions

_____

_____

_____

_____

_____

Postpartum Help

For: _____Due on:_____

Name & Phone #   Offer: meal/errand/babysit/chores/other

Thank You Kindly!

Postpartum Depression Symptoms

Baby Blues	Postpartum Depression (+ Baby Blues symptoms)	Postpartum Psychosis (+ Depression symptoms)
Physical		
lack of sleep	headaches	refusal to eat
tired after sleep	numbness, tingling in limbs	frantic, excessive energy
no energy	chest pains, heart palpitations	inability to stop activity
appetite loss or cravings	hyperventilating	
Mental		
anxiety and worry	despondence or despair	extreme confusion
great concern over physical changes	feelings of inadequacy	loss of memory
confusion and nervousness	inability to cope	incoherence
not feeling like self	hopelessness/powerlessness	bizarre hallucinations
lack of confidence	consumed with concern over baby's health	
sadness	impaired concentration or memory	
feeling overwhelmed	loss of normal interests	
	loss of interest in sex	
	thought of suicide	
	strange thoughts/fantasies	
	feelings of shame, embarrassment, or guilt	
Behavior/Reactions		
crying more than usual	extreme or unusual behavior	suspiciousness
hyperactivity or excitability	panic attacks	irrational statements
oversensitivity/ feelings hurt easily	anxiety	preoccupation with trivia
irritability with everyone	hostile or easily angered	
lack of feelings for the baby	new fears or phobias	
	wanting to be alone	
	hallucinations	
	nightmares	
	extreme guilt	
	no feelings for the baby	
	overconcern for the baby	
	anger towards the baby	
	feeling out of control/like "going crazy"	

Postpartum Depression - Questions to Consider

Postpartum depression can be a serious problem. Even if you have never been depressed before, it could happen to you.

Have you thought of harming yourself or your baby more than once? If you have, you need to get help right away.

Even if you haven't had those thoughts, you might still be headed for depression. Ask yourself these questions:

- Do you have persistent sleep problems?
- Do you feel like staying in bed all day?
- Do you often feel overwhelmed?
- Do you feel moody or depressed or cry often?
- Do you feel inadequate or feel like a failure?
- Are you much more irritable or nervous than usual?
- Do you feel like you don't care about anything?
- Do you worry about the baby for no good reason?
- Have you ever considered leaving the baby somewhere?

If you answer yes to more than two or three of these questions, you need to get professional help. Depression is a serious condition, and it's not something you should take chances with.

Chapter 12
Creating Your Own Birth Vision

Dear Readers,

Now that you've had a chance to read the past 11 chapters, you should feel better prepared to create your own birth vision. The next few pages will give you an activity and the basic information you'll need to do a birth vision that reflects your own personal philosophy (what this birth means to you), preferences (options that make sense to you), and priorities (the 3 most important of all choices listed). In the following pages, we've also included some birth visions from clients, so you can see how other women have chosen to communicate their wishes to their midwife or doctor.

Remember that the examples given are other women's visions. Maybe they'll give you some insight into how other women have felt about birth and how they wanted to approach it. You may discover an area to consider that you had never thought about before (like waiving newborn care, for example). Or you may find a line in another women's philosophy that represents exactly how you feel, but couldn't find the words to express it. You will probably also notice that everyone's priorities were different. This is what truly individualizes a birth vision. So, think long and hard about the preferences you can let go and which three really are the most crucial for you to accomplish. The examples may not sound like you at all, so be sure to reflect how you personally feel in your own birth vision. However, if you like any part of any of them, you may "borrow it" as we say in the business.

Geographically speaking, possible options and routine interventions vary greatly. Be sure to attend classes in your area, so you know what is available or what the norm is. Some care providers give you booklets with information and guidelines about how their group practices. If their routines don't appeal to you, go elsewhere. Some women talk to others who have birthed recently for suggestions or ideas. Word of mouth is always good. Other expectant parents like to take tours of hospitals or birth centers to know what's available before deciding where to give birth.

Lastly, it's important to invest time and thought and emotion into the preparation of your birth vision since it will most decidedly affect the outcome of your birth experience. A client (and doula) recently presented a birth vision to her doctor and the doctor said, "Wow, this is really short!" She liked the format, the wording, and the ease in knowing what was important to the couple. The content was discussed, questions were answered, and the doctor ended the conversation by saying that all the mom's requests were certainly "do-able." The client was very pleased with the interaction and positive results from using her birth vision as the vital tool it is meant to be. And, everyone in the room could feel the working alliance of the birth team forming. So start your first rough draft and HAPPY BIRTHING!

In the Doula spirit,

Jan and Teresa

Birth Vision Suggestions

1. Put your name(s) and the date submitted to your midwife or doctor at the top of the page. Limiting your vision to one page makes it easier for the staff to use.

2. Begin with a paragraph expressing your philosophy of birth (what it means to you, what you hope to gain from this experience, what you'd like to avoid, how you hope you'll be treated, etc.) Use the following activity pages (separately, then compare answers) to create a joint philosophy.

3. The next section can be divided into Labor, Birth, Postpartum, and Cesarean subheadings. List your preferences after considering options listed on the following page. Important issues to consider are movement and position change, fetal monitoring, IV, drugs, pushing, episiotomy, and newborn procedures.

4. Finish by highlighting your three most important issues, so your birth team can make a real effort to help you accomplish them. Discuss these with all involved before and during your birth. Take your vision with you and invite the staff to read it.

5. Remember, a birth vision is just that. It's wonderful to have goals, so you can have a sense of direction. However, it's important to be flexible and open minded so you're not set up for failure.

Happy Birthing!

Questions for Mother:

What is your personal philosophy regarding your birth?

Aside from the baby's safety, what are the three most important issues to you about your birth?

1.

2.

3.

Questions for Father:

What is your personal philosophy regarding birth?

Aside from the baby's safety, what are the three most important issues to you about your birth?

1.

2.

3.

Choices in Childbirth

Birth Site
- Home
- Birth Center
- Hospital

Healthcare Provider
- Certified Nurse Midwife
- Direct Entry Midwife
- Family Practitioner
- Obstetrician

Support during Labor
- Partner
- Friend/Family
- Doula

Hydration/Nutrition
- Light Foods
- Clear fluids/ice chips
- IV
- Heparin Lock (capped IV without tube)

Monitoring
- Doppler (used at office visits)
- External
- Internal
- Telemetric (portable & constant)
- Intermittent
- Constant

Membranes
- Rupture Naturally
- Rupture Artificially
- Amnio-infusion (putting fluid back into uterus after rupture of membranes)

Medication
- None
- Narcotics (Stadol or Nubain)
- Partial dose (¼ or ½)
- Full dose

- Epidural
  - Light (allows for movement in bed)
  - Full Dose
  - Bolus (one large dose)
  - Constant (consistent dosing)
  - Patient controlled (patient doses)
- Pitocin
  - None
  - Induction
  - Augmentation
  - Immediate Postpartum

Cesarean Birth
- Epidural
- Spinal
- General Anesthesia
- Duramorph (post-cesarean pain)
- Partner/Doula attend
- Screen lowered (to see baby at birth)
- Canula or oxygen mask
- Arm free to touch and hold baby

Pushing
- Physiologic (woman-directed)
- Directed (staff-centered)

Cord
- Cut after stops pulsing
- Cut immediately
- Cord blood collection

Episiotomy
- Avoid
- Spontaneous Separation (tear)
- Episiotomy

Postpartum Baby Care
- Eye Treatment
  - Waive
  - Postpone (until after bonding & breastfeeding)
  - Immediate

- Vitamin K
  - Waive
  - Postpone
  - Immediate

- Circumcision
  - None
  - Postpone (several days)

- Location
  - Rooming In
  - Nursery

- Feeding
  - Breastfeeding
  - Sugar Water
  - Pacifier
  - Formula

- Additional Considerations:
  - What to wear – own clothes/ hospital gown)
  - Environment – music, lighting, temperature
  - Privacy – knock first, close door, curtain drawn
  - Position changes & movement
  - Use of Hydrotherapy – shower, Jacuzzi, tub
  - Birthing ball & other tools
  - Photos/Video
  - Who cuts Cord & announces sex
  - Sibling Present/Visitation
  - Visitors – immediate/postpone /at home
  - Baby book for footprints, recorder for first cry

BIRTH VISION EXAMPLES
Birth Vision for a First Birth

Elizabeth and Nicholas' Birth Vision

We believe that birth is a natural process, and should involve as few interventions as possible. For our birth, we would like to have my mother and my doula present through the process. We would like to be informed about any procedures before they happen and given input into all decisions if possible. We consider this a family event and would prefer people knock before entering and respect our privacy if we ask for time alone.

LABOR:

I want to go into labor naturally, and progress without pitocin for as long as medically possible. I would like to be as mobile as possible during labor, free to walk, change position, and use hydrotherapy. I would prefer the telemetric monitoring for as often as monitoring is required by the hospital. **I hope to avoid an epidural, and prefer a partial dose of Nubain if I require assistance with the pain.** If required for antibiotics, I prefer a hep lock to an IV.

PUSHING:

I want to push in whatever position I feel most comfortable in. I would like the mirror available for viewing and to be given the option of touching the baby when he crowns. I'd like to avoid an episiotomy if medically possible.

IMMEDIATE POST PARTUM:

We would like all non-emergency treatments (vitamin K, bath, etc.) delayed until after the first hour. I would like to hold and breastfeed as soon as possible after the birth (kangaroo care). We do NOT want our son circumcised. We would like to waive the eye treatment. We would like to have private bonding time immediately after the birth limited to our family.

IN THE EVENT OF A CESAREAN BIRTH:

We would like to be given time to make the decision and as much information as possible. I would like to have an arm free to hold the baby immediately. I prefer to have the nasal tubes to the mask for oxygen. Please allow my husband and doula to be in the room. I'd still like to have kangaroo care if medically possible.

Birth Vision for a Second Birth

Birth Vision for Dana & Philip

Birth Philosophy

We believe that birthing process is a life-altering event for parents that can set the emotional tone for the first interactions with our new baby! After having such a positive birth experience delivering our first child, we are entering into preparing for the birth of our second child with positivity and much anticipation. We hope to use the same strategies that served us so well previously – allowing Dana to listen and instinctively respond to her body's signals and having the parents be well-informed about the birthing process in order to participate in decision making. We realize that a birth vision is not set in stone, and that while it is important to have goals, it is just as important to be open-minded and flexible. We thank you in advance for your support and cooperation with the following requests:

Labor

1. Heplock upon admission but no IV (if unnecessary)
2. Move and change positions freely
3. Make use of shower/ tub for pain relief
4. Intermittent monitoring
5. Avoidance of drugs (if requested, ½ dose of narcotics and/or walking epidural)
6. Sipping clear beverages during labor to remain hydrated
7. No pitocin to accelerate labor

Vaginal Birth

1. Upright delivery position
2. Avoid episiotomy
3. Doula to take photographs

Cesarean Birth

1. To be awake and aware
2. To have partner and Doula attend

Postpartum

1. Baby to mother after delivery
2. Husband to cut umbilical cord after it stops pulsing
3. Baby to breast within first hour
4. IV fluids
5. Nurses aware if Dana did not have epidural to adjust pressure used when pushing on uterus
6. Check for anemia (problem after birth of first child)

Three most important issues:

1. To have a medication-free birth and to use pain relief strategies, such as walking, changing positions, use of warm water as needed.
2. To remain informed about progress of labor and health of baby as to contribute to any medical decisions that arise.
3. To have the nursing staff aware and sensitive to my pain threshold during all postpartum checks, particularly in the case of a medication-free birth.

Birth Vision for a Planned Cesarean

Tamara and Allen's Birth Vision

We realize that the birth of our son will be a cesarean birth. We would like to make our birth as family-centered as we can. This is a very important day for our family, which we will remember always.

Birth

We would like to have our **doula present** with my husband and me during the cesarean. I would also like her to be there to assist me with the spinal. She has been working with us to prepare for this experience and keeps us calm. I would like to listen to ocean sounds that I provide. I would like to have one arm free to touch my son after he is given to my husband to hold. I would like for someone to be able to **take a few pictures of my son being born** and immediately after his birth as well. I prefer to have a nasal canula during the birth. I prefer to have spinal anesthesia, if appropriate. I request **double stitches to improve my chances of a VBAC later.**

Recovery & Postpartum

The first hour after birth is very important to us and as long as my son is healthy and not in distress, we would like this time to hold him, start breastfeeding and bond with him, and **not be separated from him during my recovery period.**

Our doula will stay with us through recovery and to the postpartum room to help with breastfeeding. We plan to have our son room in with us. He should not be given any supplemental formula.

Birth Vision for Induction of Labor

Alicia and Robert's Birth Vision

This is my new birth vision since I am 10 days past my due date and have been scheduled for an induction. We have tried natural methods to bring on labor, but they don't seem to be working. We hope your medical approach is successful. We were really hoping for an intervention free birth, but things have changed. We still hope to use as few interventions as possible. We may not have many options, but please consider these requests. Thank you very much.

Labor: cervidil first to ready the cervix, then slow pitocin protocol, **turn pitocin off if possible** and break water last, portable monitoring if available, hydrotherapy if possible, an epidural if it gets long or hard

Birth: Let epidural wear off for pushing, **let me labor down if not feeling urges**, upright position to bring baby down, position of my choosing for birth, tear vs. episiotomy

Postpartum: I want to announce the sex, Dad cuts cord after pulsing, apgars done in our arms if possible, **nurse in first half hour**, avoid baby care until after bonding and breastfeeding

Cesarean: Dad and doula there, keep us informed, photos ASAP, hold baby to bond, breastfeed in recovery, no separation from my baby if possible

Birth Vision for a VBAC

Mary and Irving's Birth Vision

Our first birth was a cesarean. I could not dilate past 6 centimeters, so they called it failure to progress. This time, we have chosen you as our care providers and birth team because we feel with your help we can succeed instead of fail. We are hoping to attain our vision of a vaginal birth after cesarean. We feel that believing in the process and being invested in the preparation will help us to accomplish our VBAC. We understand that it may not be possible and are open to following your guidance when medically indicated. Thank you for assisting us in welcoming our little boy into this world.

Labor: Portable monitoring, heparin lock, **no pain medicine unless requested**, want to be mobile and labor as "naturally" as possible

Birth: Choose my way of pushing, **avoid an episiotomy and tearing if possible**

Postpartum: Dad to cut cord, cord blood collection, **nurse as soon as possible**, waive eye treatment and vitamin K shot (no circumcision)

Cesarean: Dad and doula there, **as family-centered as possible**

Birth Vision for a Couple Who Had Miscarriages and IVF

Renée and David's Birth Vision

It's taken us a long time to get pregnant and then maintain a pregnancy, so this baby is very special to us. We are older parents, but this is still new to us. We are looking for not only good care from you, but guidance as well. How the baby gets here is not as important as having a healthy baby. We've chosen extra support to help us feel like we have done everything we can to have a successful birth. Thank you for all your past care. We really appreciate your continued support of us. Here are our preferences:

Labor: <u>frequent monitoring (to keep track of the baby),</u> IV if I get tired, drugs only when it's safe for the baby, don't offer an epidural—I will ask (I am open to an epidural)

Birth: Comfortable position, <u>no episiotomy unless baby needs extra room to come out</u>

Postpartum: Dad cuts cord and announces baby's sex, we are collecting cord blood. Apgars on my chest, postpone any baby care as long as possible, <u>don't separate mom and baby</u>, breastfeed within an hour, if our baby is healthy we would like some <u>undisturbed time alone to bond—just the three of us</u>, rooming in

Cesarean: Dad and doula, mirror to watch baby coming out, Dad to warmer, photos right away, don't separate mom and baby

Birth Vision for Twins

Birth Vision for Sarah and Ted

Even though twins run in our family, we were surprised that we were having two babies at one time! The most important thing to us is that they get as close to full term as possible. Other twins in our family have been a good size and even born vaginally. **That is our ultimate vision – twins born vaginally.** Please help us in any way you can to achieve that end. We understand that I am considered more high risk, but I'd like to be treated as low risk as possible. Thank you. We have highlighted preferences that mean the most to us.

Labor – **turn monitoring off for bathroom breaks**, IV on arm vs. hand, low dose of narcotics or light epidural maybe

Birth – sidelying pushing, avoid episiotomy, mirror to watch the births

Postpartum: **hold babies ASAP, try nursing right away**, baby care ok but after trying to nurse please

Cesarean: Dad and doula there, **tape recorder to record first cries and lots of photos**, Dad goes with babies if NICU is required

Birth Vision for Mom Who Has a History of Sexual Abuse

Birth Vision for Celeste and Bill

This birth vision is our way of communicating what is important to us. Thank you for reading this and discussing our wishes with us. Being proactive is our way of making sure our choices are known. My privacy is very important to me, as well as limiting the number of people that I interact with. I prefer no male doctors, nurses, residents, or students, and want as few internal exams as possible. I want to be informed whenever anyone will be touching me and I want their touch to be gentle. Here are my birth requests:

Labor: Up and moving, position changes, use ball and water, little or no drugs, little monitoring, IV only if necessary, prefer a hep lock, please knock before entering room

Birth: Semi-reclining position, grunting technique, no episiotomy hopefully, no extra observers

Postpartum: **Have my baby skin-to-skin right away**, baby shot and eye care later, breastfeeding help from my doula, **only rooming in** pediatrician checks in our room, please don't give our room number out to callers

Cesarean: Spinal preferred, sutures vs. clamps if possible, **Dad and doula both there,** Mom holds baby during repair with assistance

Bibliography

American Academy of Pediatrics. (1998). *Caring for Your Baby and Young Child Birth to Age 5*. New York: Bantam Books.

Bertram, L. (2000). *Choosing Waterbirth*. Charlottesville (VA): Hampton Roads Publishing Company, Inc.

Biancuzzo, M. 2003. *Breastfeeding the Newborn: Clinical Strategies for Nurses*. Saint Louis, MO: Mosby.

Cortlund, Y. Lucke, B., & Watelet, D.M. (2004). *Mother Rising: The Blessingway Journey into Motherhood*. Honeoye (NY): Seeing Stone Press.

Gaskin, I.M. (2003). *Ina May's Guide to Childbirth*. New York: A Bantam Book.

Gaskin, I.M. (1990). *Spiritual Midwifery*. Summertown (TN): The Book Publishing Company.

Genna, C.W. (2008). *Supporting Sucking Skills in Breastfeeding Infants*. Sudbury (Mass.): Jones and Bartlett.

Kitzinger, S. (1991). *Homebirth*. New York: Dorling Kindersley, Inc.

Kitzinger, S. (2000). *Rediscovering Birth*. New York: Pocket Books.

Kitzinger, S. (1996). *The Complete Book of Pregnancy and Childbirth*. New York: Alfred A. Knopf.

Klaus, M.H., Kennell, J.H., & Klaus, P.H. (2002). *The Doula Book*. Cambridge, MA: Perseus Books Group.

Klaus, M.H., Kennell, J.H., & Klaus, P.H. (1996). *Bonding*. Reading, MA: Addison-Wesley.

Korte, D. (1997). *The VBAC Companion*. Boston: The Harvard Common Press.

La Leche League International. (2001). *The Breastfeeding Answer Book*. Schaumburg, IL: La Leche League International.

La Leche League International. (1997). *The Womanly Art of Breastfeeding*. Schaumburg, IL: La Leche League International.

Lieberman, A.B. (1992). *Easing Labor Pain*. Boston: The Harvard Common Press.

Newman, J. & Pitman, T. (2000). *The Ultimate Breastfeeding Book of Answers*. Roseville, CA: Prima Publishing.

Odent, M. (1984). *Birth Reborn Second Edition*. Medford, NJ: Birth Works Press.

Perez, P., & Snedeker, C. (2000). *Special Women*. Johnson, VT: Cutting Edge Press.

Perez, P. (1999). *The Nuturing Touch at Birth*. Johnson, VT: Cutting Edge Press.

Sears, W. (1999). *Nighttime Parenting*. Schaumburg, IL: La Leche League International.

Sears, W., & Sears, M. (2003). *The Baby Book*. Boston: Little Brown and Company.

Sears, W., Sears, R., Sears, J., & Sears, M. (2004). *The Premature Baby Book*. New York: Little Brown and Company.

Simkin, P. (1989). *The Birth Partner*. Boston: The Harvard Common Press.

Simkin, P., Whalley, J., & Keppler, A. (1991). *Pregnancy Childbirth and the Newborn*. New York: Meadowbrook Press.

Simkin, P., & Ancheta, R. (2005). *The Labor Progress Handbook*. Oxford, UK: Blackwell Publishing, Ltd.

Stillerman, E. (1992). *Mother massage*. New York: Dell Publishing.

Glossary of Helpful Terms

3-1-1 rule: During labor, call your care provider when your contractions are 3 minutes apart, lasting a minute, for at least an hour. If you wait for this, you are likely to be in active labor upon arrival at the birth place.

5-1-1 rule: During labor, call your care provider when your contractions are 5 minutes apart, lasting for one minute, for at least one hour.

Adrenaline: Also known as epinephrine. The "fight or flight" hormone. Adrenaline slows down labor.

Afterbirth: (see Placenta)

Amniotic fluid: The fluid surrounding the baby. It nourishes and protects the baby growing within the amniotic sac.

Amniotic sac: Also called bag of waters. The innermost sac that protects the growing baby.

Antepartum doula: A woman who supports a pregnant mother who has medical complications or simply needs help before her baby is born. The doula often helps a mother who is limited to bed rest.

Anterior positioned baby: An unborn baby whose head is down and whose face is against the mother's spine. It means that the baby is lined up ideally for the birth, with the smallest part of the head coming first.

Anus: The sphincter muscle at the end of the rectum. The opening that bowel movements come from.

Apgar scores: The brief assessment of how a newborn is doing, taken at one minute after birth and again at five minutes.

Areola: The darker skin that encircles a woman's nipples.

Back labor: Contractions where much of the pain is in the mother's lower back. Back labor is often caused by a posterior positioned baby.

Beta Strep test: (see GBS-Group Beta Strep test)

Birth doula: A specially trained and experienced woman who provides physical, emotional, spiritual, informational, and mediatorial support before, during, and after the birth.

Bloody show: A discharge of vaginal blood and mucus that is a sign of labor progressing.

Braxton-Hicks contractions: Uterine-stretching contractions that allow for the individual muscle fibers of the uterus to stretch to accommodate the growing baby. If no cervical changes occur, they are not active labor contractions.

Breaking the water (breaking the bag of water): When the bag of waters breaks on its own, it is called Spontaneous Rupture of Membranes (SROM). When a doctor or midwife breaks the bag of waters, it is called amniotomy. Once the bag of waters is ruptured, the baby must be born, usually within 24 to 48 hours or so to avoid infection.

Bulging bag of waters (or **bulging sac of waters**): Also called a forebag. When the amniotic sac holding the fluid precedes the baby's head as it comes through the cervix.

Cervical effacement: (see Effacement of cervix)

Cervix: The sphincter at the lower end of the uterus where it meets the top of the vagina. Cervical changes are the majority of the changes during the first stage of labor.

Clitoris: A female sexual organ; the visible button-like portion is located above the opening of the urethra and the vagina.

Colostrum: The first milk produced before the baby is born. Colostrum is considered to be liquid gold by lactation experts because it is high in calories and immunities and helps lower jaundice. It is the perfect first food for newborns and premature babies.

Contractions of labor: Rhythmic and periodic uterine tightenings which help to thin and dilate the cervix.

Cord prolapse: Also called umbilical-cord prolapse. A rare emergency where the umbilical cord is squeezed between the bones of the baby's head and the mother's pelvis. It can cause the baby to get little or no oxygen. If you feel the cord in the vagina, get into a knees/chest position (buttocks higher than head/shoulders) and call 9-1-1.

Dystocia of Labor: A difficult birth slowed down by one of various reasons. One common kind is shoulder dystocia when the baby doesn't fit. This often leads to a cesarean birth.

Effacement of cervix: The cervix thins from zero % effacement (thick) to 100% effaced (tissue paper thin). Most of the effacement happens during labor, some happens in the weeks leading up to labor.

Effleurage: Massage using long, flowing strokes.

Endorphins: "Feel-good" chemicals produced in the pituitary gland and hypothalamus and released during labor, which help a woman cope with contraction pain.

Engagement: The baby dropping into the pelvic opening.

Epidural: Regional anesthesia placed in the space around the spine through a catheter.

Episiotomy: A cut through the skin and muscle of the perineum to enlarge the vagina for birth.

Fallopian tubes: Very thin tubes leading from the ovaries into the uterus. The ovum travels through them into the uterus.

Fetal heart tones: The baby's heartbeat as monitored before birth. It should be within a range of 120-160 heartbeats per minute.

Fetal monitoring: Monitoring used to make sure the baby inside you is healthy. Doppler monitoring is the external monitor the doctor or midwife uses at office visits and can use during labor. The external belt monitor is often used during labor either continuously or with breaks when the belt is off. The internal monitor is placed inside the uterus, and the electric lead is strapped to the leg and into the machine. Having an internal monitor usually means the mother is in bed for the rest of the birth.

Finger glide: A massage technique doulas often use, also called a nerve stroke. As the contraction is ending, the massager drags her fingers right down the body part where she began.

Forceps delivery: A delivery in which the practitioner uses forceps (a tool that looks like salad tongs) to help extract the baby. Most practitioners prefer to use vacuum extraction or cesarean delivery instead of forceps today.

Gate Control Theory: A theory of pain perception that says non-pain sensations can help block the sensation of pain. When the skin is stimulated by touch, massage, pressure, vibration, warmth, cold, or water during labor, for example, you will feel less pain from the contraction. The gate control theory kicks in and reduces the amount of pain you feel from the contraction traveling along deeper nerve pathways to get to the brain. After receiving messages from the skin, the brain begins assimilating those stimuli. So by the time the contraction pain arrives, the brain is busy - a gate drops and less pain gets in.

GBS—Group Beta Strep test: GBS is a bacterium that can cause pneumonia and meningitis in newborns. These bacteria can also colonize the intestines and the female reproductive tract, increasing the risk for premature rupture of membranes and transmission to the infant. Women are often tested for GBS between 35 and 37 weeks of their pregnancy. Women who test positive can be given antibiotics during labor, which will usually prevent transmission to the infant.

Heparin lock or Hep lock: An entrance to a vein that is established but is capped off. If an IV is needed, a catheter can be inserted into the hep lock and fluids can be given to the mother.

Hydrotherapy: Any use of water during labor, such as a Jacuzzi tub, bath, shower or sponge/hand/foot bath to relax the mom and ease her labor.

Induction of labor: Forcing labor to start for some medical reason. Medical inductions can include the use of a cervical ripener and a pitocin drip. Lower-tech inductions include nipple stimulation, induction massage, or other remedies approved by your care provider.

Involution: Contractions of the uterus after birth that clamp down on the wound left when the placenta pulled away. The process takes several days and eventually restores the uterus to its former size. Breastfeeding helps with involution.

Kegel exercise: A pelvic-floor-strengthening exercise that not only reduces incontinence, but also prepares your "bottom" for birth. By tightening and then relaxing the figure 8 of muscles that surround the vagina and rectum, you make the area healthier and better conditioned to do the work associated with birthing.

La Leche League: The internationally recognized non-profit support group for breastfeeding mothers. A source of breastfeeding information, help, and camaraderie.

Labia: The lips of the vagina, which are on either side of the vulva.

Labor contractions: (see Contractions of labor)

Labor induction: (see Induction of Labor)

Lightening: As your body prepares for birth, the baby drops lower and there is more room between your breasts and your pregnant belly.

Lochia: A postpartum vaginal discharge that can contain blood clots and mucus. It can last 3-6 weeks after birth and gets lighter in color as it decreases then stops.

Mastitis: A breast infection, usually in the duct, with redness, tenderness and flu-like symptoms.

Mature milk: The milk which comes in after 3 to 5 days of nursing. It takes the place of colostrum. It is still high in immunities and the very best milk for your baby.

Meconium: The baby's first stool that looks almost black and is sticky, odorless, and sterile.

Membrane sweep: (see Stripping of membranes)

Montgomery glands: Small bumps on the areola around the nipple that keeps it clean and moist during lactation.

Mucus plug: An accumulation of mucus within the cervix to further protect the baby from infection. Losing it sometimes means labor is close. You can tell you've lost your mucus plug if you see something that looks like mucus with strands of pink, red or brown in it.

Nipple stimulation: Stimulating the nipple with gentle massage, warmth, sucking, or pumping to encourage the release of oxytocin to begin or strengthen contractions.

Non-stress test: A period of fetal monitoring while still pregnant to assess the baby's health while not under the stress of labor.

Nuchal cord: An umbilical cord that wraps around the baby's neck.

Oxytocin: A hormone. Released during labor, it causes contractions; released during nursing, it causes the flow of milk.

Perineal massage: A massage of the perineum before the birth to help with vaginal elasticity.

Perineum: The skin and muscle between the female vagina and rectum.

Physiologic pushing: A woman-centered way of pushing the baby out where the mother determines her position, placement of legs and arms, breathing, and pushing technique.

Pitocin: An artificial hormone used to induce or augment labor or treat bleeding after a birth.

Placenta (afterbirth): A special organ that transfers oxygen, nutrients, hormones, and waste products between mother and baby.

Posterior-positioned baby: A baby who is facing the mother's front, so its hard, bony head is pressing against her spine, causing back pain and back labor.

Postpartum depression: Depression after giving birth that lasts longer than the blues. Postpartum depression is a serious disease that can hamper your ability to take care of your baby and live a normal life.

Postpartum doula: A specially trained, experienced woman who provides support, guidance, and care for a new family once the baby is born.

Pre-eclampsia: A disease associated with pregnancy with symptoms of high blood pressure, swelling, and protein in the urine.

Prolactin: The hormone that causes milk production.

Prostaglandins: Substances in many tissues that affect reproductive function and can be used for cervical ripening.

Rebozo: A shawl used by Mexican midwives during labor for the mother's comfort, and to help with positioning the baby and delivery.

Round ligaments: Two of the 10 ligaments that stabilize the uterus within the pelvis.

Stripping of membranes: Also called sweeping of membranes. A finger is inserted into a partially dilated cervix and a sweeping motion is used to separate the amniotic sac from the uterus. The stripping can cause a release of prostaglandins to start labor.

Super Kegel exercise: Holding the pelvic floor muscles in and up for a count of 20 (which is longer than for regular Kegel exercises) to condition the area better for birth. See Kegel exercise.

Telemetric monitoring: Portable constant monitoring that enables the mother to move better.

Terminal meconium: The release of its first bowel movement as the baby is being born.

Three stages of labor: First stage, cervical dilation; second stage, birth of the baby; third stage, delivery of the placenta.

Vacuum extraction: The use of a vacuum instrument to help with delivery of a baby. If a mother cannot push the baby all the way to delivery, some practitioners will try a vacuum extraction before moving to a cesarean.

VBAC: Vaginal birth after cesarean.

Vernix: A protective white, waxy, cheesy-looking coating on newborns that protects their skin while in the uterus.

Author Bios

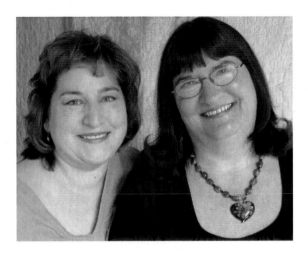

Teresa F. Bailey, J.D., M.L.S., CD(DONA), LLL Leader, is a lawyer who has worked for a decade as a doula in Pittsburgh. She works closely with Jan Mallak in the "Heart & Hands"SM doula group. In addition to her doctorate in law and her doula training, she has a master's degree in library science and a bachelor's degree in philosophy and mathematics. She is also a leader in La Leche League, the international breastfeeding support organization. Her unique combination of skills gives her a different perspective on her work from what most doulas can offer. As a lawyer who gave up her law career to work as a doula, she brings a single-minded dedication to her work that shows through in everything she writes. She lives in inner-city Pittsburgh with her husband Christopher and their nine-year-old son, Simon.

Jan S. Mallak, 2LAS,ICCE-CD-CPD-IAT,CD-PCD(DONA), CPD(CAPPA) has 30 years in the baby business. She is an internationally certified childbirth educator and is certified as a birth and postpartum doula by several organizations. Jan is also an ICEA approved trainer as well as a DONA approved birth doula trainer. She is also the founder and coordinator of "Heart & Hands"SM Doula Service, which is the oldest, largest (since 1995) and most comprehensive doula agency in Western Pennsylvania. Jan has been published many times, is a well known speaker, provides birth consulting and is also an artist. She is lovingly supported by her husband, Frank, of 37 years, grown children, Frankie, Heather, Dror and now, her first grandchild, Zeev.

Index